Dreaming of Youth

The Role of Sleep in Prolonging Health and Vitality

A short introduction by The HealthSpan Institute

Dreaming of Youth:
The Role of Sleep in Prolonging Health and Vitality

ISBN: 9798869616050

Copyright © 2023 Wellness Press

All rights reserved. No part of this publication may be reproduced, stored on a retrieval system, or transmitted, in any form or by any means, electronic, mechanical, photocopying, microfilming, recording or otherwise, without written permission from the publisher.

Printed in the United States of America

Contents

Chapter 2:
Sleep and Aging

Chapter 3:
Sleep's Role in Physical Health

Chapter 4:
Mental Health and Cognitive Function

Chapter 5:
Sleep Disorders and Their Impact on Aging

Chapter 6:
Enhancing Sleep Quality

Chapter 7:
Technological Advances in Sleep Science

Chapter 8:
Cultural and Societal Perspectives on Sleep

Conclusion

Appendix A:
Resources for further reading and research

Appendix B:
Sleep assessment tools and questionnaires

Appendix C:
Directory of sleep clinics and experts

Preface

Introduction to the Book's Theme and Purpose

In the tapestry of life, each thread of health and wellness is intricately woven, with sleep being one of its most fundamental strands. "Dreaming of Youth: The Role of Sleep in Prolonging Health and Vitality" is born out of a deep exploration into this often underestimated aspect of our lives. This book aims to unravel the mysteries of sleep and its profound impact on aging, unraveling how the elixir of restful nights can be the key to a more vibrant, healthier, and longer life.

The journey of this book is a quest for understanding, a pilgrimage into the heart of nocturnal rejuvenation. Here, sleep is not just an act of nightly repose but a powerful agent of health and vitality. It's a force that shapes our days, dictates our health, and ultimately, influences the trajectory of our aging. This work is grounded in the belief that in the realm of deep and restful sleep lies the secret to preserving youthfulness, both in body and spirit.

The narrative of sleep as a cornerstone of health is as old as time, yet it's a tale that's often overshadowed by more conspicuous health advice. In a world that glorifies busyness and undervalues rest, "Dreaming of Youth" seeks to restore the balance. It challenges the modern narrative that associates rest with idleness and redefines sleep as an active, vital process that rejuvenates and repairs the body and mind. This book is an invitation to rekindle a friendship with one's own sleep patterns and to recognize the night as a healer.

Through the pages of this book, readers will embark on a journey that begins with the science of sleep. Understanding the complex ballet of brain waves and the symphony of hormones that orchestrate our sleep cycles is the first step towards appreciating sleep's role in our lives. This journey is not just about the quantity of sleep but the quality, delving into the nuances that transform mere rest into a rejuvenative experience.

As we delve deeper, the book explores the symbiotic relationship between sleep and aging. How does our sleep change as we age, and more intriguingly, how can our sleep affect the way we age? This exploration is not just limited to the physical realm but extends to the mental and emotional landscapes as well. We'll discover how the threads of sleep weave through the fabric of our mental wellbeing, influencing everything from our mood to our cognitive abilities.

In a world rife with sleep disorders and nocturnal unrest, "Dreaming of Youth" doesn't shy away from the darker side of sleep. Insomnia, sleep apnea, and other disorders not only disrupt our nights but also cast long shadows over our health and longevity. This book aims to be a beacon of hope, illuminating the path towards understanding and overcoming these nocturnal challenges. It's about empowering individuals with knowledge and practical strategies to reclaim the sanctity of their sleep.

But this book's vision goes beyond individual struggles and triumphs. It recognizes sleep as a societal issue, affected and influenced by cultural, economic, and technological forces. In a world where screens invade our bedrooms and work encroaches upon our rest, understanding these external forces is crucial. "Dreaming of Youth" seeks to spark a conversation about how society views and values sleep, advocating for a cultural shift that places sleep at the forefront of public health.

At its core, "Dreaming of Youth" is a celebration of sleep and a recognition of its role in our quest for longevity and vitality. It's a guide, a companion, and a source of enlightenment for those seeking to harness the restorative power of sleep. This book aspires to be a turning point in how we perceive and prioritize our nightly rest. It aims to shift the paradigm from viewing sleep as a mere necessity to recognizing it as a powerful ally in our journey towards a healthier, more vibrant life.

As you turn the pages, you'll find not just facts and research, but stories, experiences, and insights that bring the world of sleep to life. From the latest scientific discoveries to age-old wisdom, from practical tips to philosophical musings, this book is a mosaic of everything sleep represents in our quest for health and youthfulness.

In this fast-paced world, where the night often becomes a mere extension of the day, "Dreaming of Youth" is an invitation to pause, reflect, and embrace the night's embrace. It's a call to journey back to the essence of restful, restorative sleep, and in doing so, rediscover the fountain of youth that resides within each of us. Welcome to a journey of nocturnal revelation, a journey towards dreaming of youth.

Brief Personal or Anecdotal Evidence Highlighting the Transformative Power of Sleep

In the narrative of human health and vitality, sleep often emerges as a silent yet powerful protagonist. The transformative power of sleep is not just a subject of scientific inquiry but also a theme resonant in countless personal stories and anecdotes. These narratives, woven from the fabric of individual experiences, bring to light the profound impact that sleep can have on our lives.

One such story is that of Anna, a middle-aged professional who grappled with the pressures of a demanding career and a bustling family life. For years, Anna considered sleep as nothing more than a necessary pause, a reluctant concession to her body's limitations. Her nights were short, often interrupted, and her days were marked by a persistent fog of fatigue. It wasn't until a routine medical check-up revealed the onset of hypertension and heightened stress levels that Anna began to reconsider her approach to sleep.

Motivated by concern for her health and encouraged by her doctor, Anna embarked on a journey to transform her sleep habits. It began with small changes: setting a regular bedtime, creating a relaxing bedtime routine, and making her bedroom a sanctuary for sleep. The transformation was gradual but profound. Over weeks and months, Anna began to notice a remarkable change. Her energy levels increased, her mood stabilized, and she found a new sense of clarity and focus in her work. Sleep, which once was a begrudged necessity, had become her most potent ally in health and vitality.

Then there's the story of David, a retired veteran, whose experience with sleep was marked by the nightmares and restlessness of post-traumatic stress disorder (PTSD). For David, the night was a time of turmoil, not tranquility. His journey with sleep was a battle, one where the demons of his past clashed with his quest for peace in the present. The turning point came with therapy and a structured approach to sleep, which included mindfulness practices and sleep hygiene techniques. As his sleep improved, so did his mental health. The nightmares receded, giving way to more peaceful nights, and in turn, more joyful days. David's story is a testament to the healing power of sleep, not just for the body, but for the mind and soul.

Another compelling anecdote comes from the life of Sarah, a young athlete whose dreams of competing at a high level were almost derailed by chronic fatigue and injury. Sarah's rigorous training schedule and academic commitments left little room for rest, and sleep was often an afterthought. It was only after a conversation with her coach, who emphasized the role of sleep in recovery and performance, that Sarah began to rethink her approach. By prioritizing sleep, she not only saw improvements in her athletic performance but also in her academic and personal life. Sleep became her secret weapon, a source of strength and resilience.

These stories, diverse in their backgrounds and experiences, converge on a common theme: the transformative power of sleep. They underscore the fact that sleep is not a passive state of inactivity but a dynamic process of restoration and rejuvenation. Through these narratives, we see how sleep can be a catalyst for positive change, impacting various facets of our lives.

In "Dreaming of Youth," these stories and others like them are not just anecdotes; they are evidence of the power of sleep. They serve as reminders that our nights hold the key to our days, that in our sleep lies the potential for transformation and rejuvenation. These narratives are interwoven throughout the book, providing not just context but inspiration. They serve as living proof that when we honor our need for rest, we unlock our full potential for health, vitality, and longevity.

These stories also remind us that the journey towards better sleep is deeply personal and unique. What works for one may not work for another, and the path to restful nights can be as varied as the individuals who walk it. But the underlying message is universal: respect for sleep and an understanding of its role in our lives is fundamental to our well-being.

As you delve into the pages of "Dreaming of Youth," let these stories be a source of motivation and insight. Let them be a reminder that in the realm of sleep lies untapped potential for transformation. Let them inspire you to explore your own relationship with sleep and discover its powerful impact on your journey towards health and vitality. For in these stories lies not just the power of sleep but the power within each of us to harness it.

Chapter 1: The Science of Sleep

Understanding Sleep: Its Stages and Cycles

Sleep, often perceived as a single, uniform state of rest, is in fact a complex, multifaceted process. It's a journey through various stages, each characterized by distinct patterns of brain activity and physiological changes. To fully appreciate the intricacies of sleep and its impact on our health and well-being, it's essential to delve into the understanding of its stages and cycles.

The Architecture of Sleep

Sleep is architecturally structured in cycles, each lasting about 90 to 110 minutes. These cycles are comprised of four distinct stages: three stages of Non-Rapid Eye Movement (NREM) sleep and one stage of Rapid Eye Movement (REM) sleep. As the night progresses, the composition and duration of these stages fluctuate, creating a dynamic interplay that is vital for the restorative functions of sleep.

The NREM Stages

Stage 1 (N1)

The first stage of sleep, N1, is the transition from wakefulness to sleep. It's a light sleep stage where one can be easily awakened. During this stage, muscle tone throughout the body relaxes, and brain wave patterns shift from the alpha waves characteristic of wakefulness to slower theta waves. This stage typically lasts for just a few minutes and constitutes about 5% of a typical night's sleep.

Stage 2 (N2)

Stage 2, or N2, marks the onset of true sleep. The body delves deeper into relaxation, with further reductions in heart rate and body temperature. This stage is characterized by the appearance of sleep spindles–brief bursts of rapid brain activity–and K-complexes, which are large, slow brain waves. These phenomena are thought to play a role in consolidating memories and information processing. Stage 2 sleep comprises approximately 45-55% of total sleep in adults.

Stage 3 (N3)

Often referred to as deep sleep or slow-wave sleep (SWS), stage 3 is the most restorative stage of sleep. It's characterized by delta waves, which are the slowest and highest amplitude brain waves. During this stage, the body repairs and regrows tissues, builds bone and muscle, and strengthens the immune system. Deep sleep is crucial for physical recovery and health, and it's during this stage that growth hormone is released. This stage occupies about 20% of sleep in adults but decreases with age.

The REM Stage

The final stage in the sleep cycle is REM sleep, named for the rapid and random movement of the eyes under the eyelids. This stage is markedly different from the NREM stages. Brain wave activity becomes faster, resembling that of wakefulness, and the body experiences a state of atonia, where the muscles are temporarily paralyzed. REM sleep is the stage associated with the most vivid dreams.

It's in REM sleep that significant brain activities occur, including memory consolidation and the processing of emotions. This stage is essential for cognitive functions such as learning, problem-solving, and creativity. In adults, REM sleep constitutes about 20-25% of total sleep, and its duration tends to increase in the latter half of the night.

The Cyclic Nature of Sleep

Throughout the night, we cycle through these stages multiple times. The first sleep cycle tends to have a shorter REM period, with subsequent cycles having longer REM stages. As morning approaches, NREM sleep, particularly the deep N3 stage, diminishes in favor of increased REM sleep. This cyclical pattern is regulated by the brain's internal clock and external cues like light and darkness, forming the basis of our circadian rhythms.

The Significance of Sleep Stages

Each stage of sleep serves a unique function. The NREM stages are primarily associated with physical restoration and rejuvenation, while REM sleep is crucial for brain health and emotional regulation. A disruption in the normal progression through these stages, such as in sleep disorders, can have profound impacts on both mental and physical health.

Understanding the stages of sleep is not just an academic exercise. It offers a window into the workings of our body and mind during rest. It helps us appreciate the complexity of sleep and its essential role in our overall health and well-being.

In "Dreaming of Youth," this understanding serves as a foundation for exploring the myriad ways in which sleep affects our health, mood, cognitive abilities, and even our longevity. As we unravel the mysteries of these nocturnal stages, we gain insights into how we can optimize our sleep for a healthier, more vibrant life.

The Brain During Sleep: Neurochemistry and Brain Wave Patterns

Sleep is not just a state of rest for the body; it's a dynamic and essential period of activity for the brain. Understanding the neurochemical processes and brain wave patterns during sleep is crucial to comprehending the role of sleep in health and cognition. This section of "Dreaming of Youth" delves into the fascinating world of the sleeping brain, exploring how neurochemistry and brain waves orchestrate the symphony of sleep.

The Neurochemistry of Sleep

The brain's activity during sleep is a complex interplay of neurotransmitters and hormones, each playing a specific role in regulating sleep stages and cycles. Neurotransmitters such as GABA (gamma-aminobutyric acid) and glycine promote relaxation and are pivotal in initiating sleep. They counterbalance the wakefulness-promoting neurotransmitters like norepinephrine, serotonin, and histamine.

Melatonin, often referred to as the 'sleep hormone', is produced in the pineal gland and plays a crucial role in regulating sleep-wake cycles. Its production is influenced by the circadian rhythm and external light, increasing in the evening to promote sleepiness and decreasing in the morning. Cortisol, the stress hormone, follows a reverse pattern, peaking in the early morning to promote wakefulness.

Adenosine, a neuromodulator that accumulates in the brain during waking hours, also plays a significant role. It creates a 'sleep pressure' that increases the longer we stay awake, and decreases during sleep, particularly during deep sleep. The balance and interaction of these neurochemicals are essential for the maintenance of healthy sleep patterns.

Brain Wave Patterns in Sleep

The brain's electrical activity, which can be observed through electroencephalography (EEG), varies significantly across the different stages of sleep. Brain waves, the rhythmic electrical patterns produced by the brain, change noticeably as we cycle through the stages of sleep.

Wakefulness to Stage 1 (N1) Transition

During wakefulness, the brain exhibits beta waves, which are high-frequency, low-amplitude waves associated with active, alert states. As we transition to sleep, these give way to alpha waves, indicative of a relaxed, wakeful state. The onset of Stage 1 sleep sees the emergence of theta waves, slower and higher in amplitude than alpha waves, signaling the beginning of the sleep cycle.

Stage 2 (N2) Sleep

In Stage 2 sleep, theta waves continue to dominate. This stage is characterized by two unique EEG patterns: sleep spindles and K-complexes. Sleep spindles are bursts of rapid, rhythmic brain activity that may play a role in memory consolidation and synaptic plasticity. K-complexes are single, high-amplitude waves thought to be involved in cognitive processes related to memory and also serve as a bridge to deeper stages of sleep.

Stage 3 (N3) Sleep

Deep sleep or slow-wave sleep (SWS) is marked by delta waves, the slowest and highest amplitude brain waves. These waves are considered the hallmark of Stage 3 sleep and are associated with the restoration and recovery processes of the body and brain. It is during this stage that the brain consolidates memories and information and the body undergoes physical repair and growth.

REM Sleep

REM sleep presents a unique brain wave pattern, where activity closely resembles that of an awake state. The brain waves are predominantly low-amplitude, mixed-frequency patterns similar to beta waves. This paradoxical state, where the brain is active but the body is in a state of muscle atonia (paralysis), is essential for processes related to learning, memory consolidation, and emotional processing.

The Role of Brain Waves in Sleep

Each of these brain wave patterns signifies a different phase of sleep, with distinct physiological and neurological functions. The progression through these stages and the accompanying brain wave changes are crucial for cognitive functions such as learning, memory formation, and emotional regulation. Disruptions in these patterns can lead to impaired cognitive function and have been associated with various sleep disorders.

Furthermore, the study of brain waves during sleep provides valuable insights into age-related changes in sleep patterns. For instance, the amount of deep sleep and the prevalence of delta waves decrease with age, which may contribute to age-related cognitive decline and health issues.

In conclusion, the neurochemistry and brain wave patterns during sleep reveal a world of intricate processes that are fundamental to our physical, cognitive, and emotional well-being. Understanding these patterns not only enlightens us about the science of sleep but also empowers us to make informed choices about our sleep health.

Circadian Rhythms and Their Impact on Overall Health

The concept of circadian rhythms, the natural cycles of physical, mental, and behavioral changes that follow a 24-hour cycle, is integral to understanding sleep and its extensive influence on health. These rhythms, often referred to as the body's internal clock, are not only pivotal in regulating the sleep-wake cycle but also play a significant role in various bodily functions. In "Dreaming of Youth," we explore how these rhythms shape our health and well-being.

The Nature of Circadian Rhythms

Circadian rhythms are driven by an internal biological clock, primarily located in the suprachiasmatic nucleus (SCN) in the hypothalamus of the brain. This clock is influenced by external environmental cues, most notably light, which help synchronize the rhythms to the 24-hour day-night cycle. These rhythms regulate critical functions such as sleep, hormone release, eating habits, digestion, and body temperature.

Sleep-Wake Cycle and Circadian Rhythms

The most apparent manifestation of circadian rhythms is the sleep-wake cycle. The SCN, responding to light and darkness, signals the pineal gland to secrete melatonin, a hormone that induces sleepiness, during the night. Conversely, in response to light, melatonin production is suppressed, promoting wakefulness and alertness. Disruptions in these rhythms, such as those caused by jet lag or shift work, can lead to sleep disorders, impacting overall health and well-being.

Hormonal Regulation

Circadian rhythms also govern the release of various hormones, including cortisol, the stress hormone. Cortisol levels typically peak in the early morning to help wake us up and gradually decline throughout the day. The synchronization of hormonal release with circadian rhythms is crucial for optimal body functioning. Imbalances or disruptions can lead to health issues like metabolic disorders, mood disturbances, and weakened immune response.

Metabolism and Circadian Rhythms

The body's metabolism is closely linked to circadian rhythms. These rhythms influence appetite, digestion, and the processing of fats and sugars. When the circadian rhythm is disrupted, it can lead to metabolic imbalances, contributing to obesity, diabetes, and cardiovascular diseases. A regular sleep schedule helps maintain a healthy metabolism, emphasizing the importance of synchronized circadian rhythms.

Immune System Function

Circadian rhythms also play a role in regulating the immune system. The production and activity of immune cells are timed to the body's internal clock, optimizing the body's defense mechanisms at different times of the day. Disruption of these rhythms can weaken the immune response, making the body more susceptible to infections and diseases.

Mental Health and Circadian Rhythms

There is a profound link between circadian rhythms and mental health. Irregular rhythms have been associated with various mental health disorders, including depression, bipolar disorder, and anxiety. The regulation of neurotransmitters and hormones, which are influenced by the circadian clock, plays a significant role in mood and cognitive functions.

Impact of Age on Circadian Rhythms

As we age, changes in circadian rhythms are observed. Older adults often experience advanced sleep phase syndrome, where they go to sleep early and wake up early. These changes can disrupt sleep quality and have implications for physical and mental health. Understanding and adapting to these changes are crucial for maintaining health and well-being in older age.

Lifestyle and Environmental Influences

Modern lifestyle choices and environmental factors can significantly impact circadian rhythms. Exposure to artificial light, especially blue light from screens, can disrupt the natural sleep-wake cycle. Similarly, irregular sleep schedules, caffeine consumption, and stress can interfere with the body's internal clock. Maintaining a routine that aligns with natural circadian rhythms is essential for optimal health.

Strategies for Maintaining Healthy Circadian Rhythms

- **Regular Sleep Schedule:** Sticking to a consistent sleep-wake schedule even on weekends helps to keep circadian rhythms stable.
- **Light Exposure:** Exposure to natural light during the day and minimizing light exposure, especially blue light, in the evening can enhance circadian regulation.
- **Diet and Exercise:** Timely meals and regular physical activity can reinforce the natural rhythms of the body.

In conclusion, circadian rhythms are a fundamental aspect of our biological functioning, deeply intertwined with sleep and overall health. Disruptions in these rhythms can have far-reaching impacts on physical, mental, and emotional well-being. By understanding and respecting these natural cycles, as detailed in "Dreaming of Youth," we can optimize our sleep and bolster our health, contributing to a more youthful and vibrant life.

Chapter 2:
Sleep and Aging

How Sleep Patterns Change as We Age

As we traverse the journey of life, one of the most significant yet subtle changes we experience is in our sleep patterns. Aging brings about a transformation in how we sleep, both in terms of quality and quantity. This section of "Dreaming of Youth" delves into the nuances of how sleep evolves with age and the implications of these changes on our overall well-being.

The Evolution of Sleep in the Aging Process

Changes in Sleep Architecture

As we age, the architecture of our sleep undergoes noticeable alterations. Older adults often experience a decrease in the amount of deep sleep or slow-wave sleep (SWS), characterized by delta brain waves. This stage of sleep is crucial for physical restoration and memory consolidation. The reduction in SWS means that sleep becomes lighter and more fragmented, making older adults more prone to awakenings during the night.

Shift in Circadian Rhythms

Another significant change is the shift in circadian rhythms. Many older adults tend to experience advanced sleep phase syndrome, where they feel sleepy earlier in the evening and wake up earlier in the morning. This shift can disrupt the alignment with the traditional 24-hour day-night cycle, leading to challenges in maintaining social and professional commitments.

Reduction in REM Sleep

The amount of Rapid Eye Movement (REM) sleep, a phase associated with vivid dreaming and important for cognitive functions like memory and learning, also tends to decrease with age. This reduction can have implications for cognitive health and emotional regulation.

Factors Contributing to Changes in Sleep Patterns

Physical Health Issues

Various health issues common in older age, such as arthritis, back pain, and respiratory problems, can interfere with sleep. Pain and discomfort can make it difficult to find a comfortable sleeping position, leading to frequent awakenings and restless nights.

Psychological Factors

Mental health issues like depression and anxiety, which are more prevalent in the elderly, can adversely affect sleep quality. Worries about health, financial security, and social changes can lead to increased stress and sleep disturbances.

Medications

Many older adults take medications that can impact sleep. Some drugs may interfere with the natural sleep cycle, while others might induce drowsiness during the day, disrupting the regular sleep-wake pattern.

Lifestyle and Environmental Changes

Retirement and changes in social routines can lead to less structured days, affecting the regularity of sleep schedules. Additionally, reduced exposure to natural light and decreased physical activity can negatively impact sleep.

The Impact of Age-Related Sleep Changes

Cognitive Impairment

A decrease in quality sleep, particularly in deep and REM sleep, can lead to cognitive impairments. Memory consolidation, learning, and problem-solving abilities can be adversely affected.

Physical Health

Disturbed sleep patterns can exacerbate age-related physical health issues, including weakened immunity, increased risk of heart disease, and metabolic imbalances.

Emotional Well-being

Poor sleep can impact mood, leading to increased irritability, depression, and a general decline in emotional well-being.

Adapting to Sleep Changes in Aging

Understanding and adapting to these changes in sleep patterns are key to maintaining health and well-being in older age.

Establishing a Regular Sleep Schedule

Maintaining a consistent sleep schedule helps regulate the body's internal clock and improves sleep quality. Going to bed and waking up at the same time every day can reinforce the natural circadian rhythm.

Creating a Sleep-Conducive Environment

A quiet, dark, and cool sleeping environment can promote better sleep. Comfortable bedding and minimizing noise and light disturbances can make a significant difference.

Diet and Exercise

A balanced diet and regular physical activity can positively impact sleep quality. Avoiding heavy meals, caffeine, and alcohol close to bedtime is also beneficial.

Stress Management and Relaxation Techniques

Practices like meditation, deep breathing, and gentle yoga can reduce stress and promote relaxation, making it easier to fall and stay asleep.

Seeking Medical Advice

It's important for older adults to discuss their sleep concerns with healthcare providers. A medical evaluation can help identify and treat underlying health issues or medication side effects that may be affecting sleep.

Conclusion

Sleep patterns naturally change as we age, and these changes can have significant effects on our health and quality of life. By understanding these alterations and adapting our lifestyles accordingly, we can mitigate some of the negative impacts and maintain our health and vitality into older age.

The Relationship Between Sleep Quality and Aging

The intertwining of sleep quality and aging is a complex and multi-faceted phenomenon. While aging invariably brings about changes in sleep patterns, the quality of sleep we maintain as we age can have profound implications on the aging process itself. In "Dreaming of Youth," we explore this intricate relationship, shedding light on how sleep quality affects aging and, conversely, how the aging process impacts sleep quality.

The Bidirectional Nature of Sleep and Aging

Impact of Sleep Quality on Aging

Sleep quality is a critical factor in determining overall health and well-being, particularly as we age. Good sleep quality is associated with various positive health outcomes, including enhanced cognitive function, better emotional balance, and a stronger immune system. In contrast, poor sleep quality can accelerate certain aging processes, contributing to cognitive decline, increased susceptibility to chronic diseases, and diminished physical capabilities.

Aging's Effect on Sleep Quality

As we age, physiological changes in the body and brain can affect sleep architecture, leading to alterations in sleep patterns. These changes often result in reduced sleep efficiency, increased sleep fragmentation, and a decrease in deep sleep stages. This can create a cycle where aging affects sleep quality, which in turn, has further implications on the aging process.

Physiological and Cognitive Aspects

Cognitive Health

There's a significant correlation between sleep quality and cognitive health in older adults. Sleep, especially deep and REM sleep, plays a critical role in memory consolidation and cognitive processing. Poor sleep quality can impair these functions, leading to faster cognitive decline and a higher risk of developing dementia-related conditions.

Physical Health

Good sleep quality is essential for physical health maintenance. It aids in the repair of cells and tissues, helps regulate metabolism, and maintains cardiovascular health. As sleep quality deteriorates with age, there is an increased risk of developing conditions like obesity, diabetes, hypertension, and heart disease.

Psychological and Emotional Dimensions

Emotional Well-being

Sleep quality directly impacts mood and emotional regulation. Chronic sleep disturbances can lead to irritability, depression, and anxiety. As people age, the ability to manage these emotional challenges can become more difficult, making the maintenance of good sleep quality even more essential for emotional well-being.

Stress and Sleep

The relationship between stress and sleep is particularly pronounced in older adults. Increased stress levels can disrupt sleep patterns, while poor sleep can enhance stress responses. This bidirectional relationship underscores the importance of managing stress to improve sleep quality, thereby positively influencing the aging process.

Lifestyle and Environmental Influences

Lifestyle Factors

Lifestyle choices such as diet, exercise, and substance use have a significant impact on sleep quality. A balanced diet, regular physical activity, and the avoidance of stimulants and alcohol can improve sleep quality, which in turn positively affects the aging process.

Environmental Factors

The sleeping environment plays a crucial role in sleep quality. Factors such as light, noise, and temperature can significantly impact sleep, especially for older adults who may have heightened sensitivity to environmental disturbances.

Strategies to Improve Sleep Quality in Aging

Regular Sleep Schedule

Maintaining a consistent sleep-wake cycle helps regulate the body's internal clock and can improve sleep quality. This regularity is especially important for older adults as it helps to counteract the effects of age-related changes in sleep patterns.

Sleep Environment Optimization

Creating a comfortable and conducive sleep environment is critical. This includes a comfortable mattress and pillows, a quiet and dark room, and an ideal room temperature.

Mindfulness and Relaxation Techniques

Practices such as meditation, deep breathing, and progressive muscle relaxation can be beneficial in improving sleep quality. These techniques help in reducing stress and promoting relaxation, aiding in better sleep.

Medical Consultation

Older adults experiencing sleep issues should consult healthcare professionals. Medical evaluation can help identify and address underlying conditions or medications affecting sleep quality.

Conclusion

The intricate relationship between sleep quality and aging is one that warrants attention and care. Good sleep quality can be a protective factor against many age-related health issues, while poor sleep can exacerbate the aging process. Understanding and addressing the factors that influence sleep quality is essential for maintaining health and vitality in older age.

Strategies to Improve Sleep in Later Years

As we advance in years, the quest for a restful night's sleep can become more challenging. The changes in sleep patterns and quality that accompany aging necessitate specific strategies tailored to this stage of life. In "Dreaming of Youth," we explore various approaches to enhance sleep in the later years, emphasizing the importance of adapting to the evolving needs of our bodies and minds.

Understanding and Adapting to Age-Related Changes

The first step in improving sleep in later years is acknowledging and understanding the changes in sleep patterns that occur with age. This includes earlier bedtimes and wake times, lighter sleep, and more frequent awakenings. Adapting lifestyle and routines to align with these changes can make a significant difference in sleep quality.

Establishing Consistent Sleep Routines

A regular sleep routine is crucial for maintaining good sleep hygiene. Going to bed and waking up at the same time every day, including weekends, can help regulate the body's internal clock and improve sleep quality. Consistency is key, even if it means adjusting schedules to suit earlier sleep and wake times.

Creating a Conducive Sleep Environment

The bedroom environment plays a pivotal role in facilitating restful sleep. It should be quiet, dark, and cool. Investing in comfortable bedding, using blackout curtains, and maintaining a comfortable room temperature can create an ideal sleeping environment. Reducing noise levels, either through the use of earplugs or sound-proofing, can also be beneficial.

Managing Diet and Nutrition

Dietary habits have a significant impact on sleep quality. It's advisable to avoid heavy meals, caffeine, and alcohol close to bedtime as they can disrupt sleep. Incorporating foods rich in magnesium and potassium, such as bananas and almonds, can promote relaxation and better sleep. Staying hydrated throughout the day, but reducing fluid intake before bedtime, can minimize nighttime awakenings for bathroom visits.

Engaging in Regular Physical Activity

Regular physical activity can greatly enhance sleep quality. Activities like walking, swimming, or light aerobic exercises, when done consistently, can help deepen sleep. However, it's important to avoid vigorous exercise close to bedtime as it can have the opposite effect.

Reducing Stress and Anxiety

Stress and anxiety can be significant barriers to restful sleep, especially in later years. Engaging in stress-reducing activities such as reading, listening to soothing music, or practicing relaxation techniques like deep breathing exercises and meditation can be helpful. Maintaining a journal to jot down worries or to-do lists before bed can also alleviate a racing mind.

Limiting Screen Time Before Bed

Exposure to blue light from screens of televisions, computers, and smartphones can interfere with the body's production of melatonin, the hormone that regulates sleep. Limiting screen time an hour before bedtime can aid in falling asleep more easily.

Mindfulness and Relaxation Techniques

Mindfulness practices and relaxation techniques can be particularly effective in improving sleep quality. Techniques such as progressive muscle relaxation, guided imagery, or gentle yoga can relax the mind and body, making it easier to drift into sleep.

Consulting Healthcare Professionals

Regular check-ups with healthcare professionals can help in identifying and addressing any underlying medical conditions that might be affecting sleep. This includes reviewing medications that may have sleep-related side effects. Seeking advice from sleep specialists or participating in sleep therapy can also provide tailored strategies to improve sleep.

Embracing Napping with Caution

While napping can be beneficial, especially when night sleep is insufficient, it's important to approach napping cautiously. Short, early afternoon naps can be refreshing, but long or late naps can interfere with nighttime sleep.

Utilizing Sleep Aids Wisely

While over-the-counter sleep aids or prescription medications can be tempting, they should be used judiciously and under medical supervision. Natural sleep aids, such as melatonin supplements, may be a safer alternative, but it's important to discuss their use with a healthcare provider.

Community and Social Engagement

Maintaining a socially active lifestyle can have positive effects on sleep. Engaging in community activities, spending time with friends and family, or participating in group exercises can promote a sense of well-being and improve sleep quality.

Conclusion

Improving sleep in later years involves a holistic approach that encompasses lifestyle, environment, diet, physical activity, and mental health. By adopting these strategies, older adults can enhance their sleep quality, contributing significantly to their overall health and well-being.

Chapter 3: Sleep's Role in Physical Health

Sleep and the Immune System: Fighting Aging and Disease

In the intricate dance of health and well-being, sleep and the immune system are closely intertwined partners. The influence of sleep on the immune system is profound, particularly in the context of aging and disease. "Dreaming of Youth" delves into how sleep serves as a foundational pillar for a robust immune system, playing a critical role in combating aging and disease.

The Symbiotic Relationship Between Sleep and Immunity

Sleep and the immune system share a symbiotic relationship where each influences and enhances the other. Adequate sleep bolsters the immune system, which in turn helps to maintain healthy sleep patterns. This relationship becomes increasingly important as we age, given the natural decline in immune function.

Boosting Immune Cell Function

During sleep, the body undergoes various processes that support immune function. Key immune cells, such as T cells and cytokines, are produced and rejuvenated during sleep. T cells are crucial for fighting off pathogens, while cytokines are involved in the immune response to inflammation and infection. Sleep enhances the ability of these cells to adhere to and attack pathogens, making sleep a critical component of immune defense.

Sleep and Vaccination Efficacy

Sleep has been shown to impact the efficacy of vaccinations. Adequate sleep following vaccination improves the body's response, leading to the production of more antibodies and a stronger immune memory. This is particularly pertinent for older adults who are often the target of vaccinations for age-related diseases.

Sleep Deprivation and Immune Function

Sleep deprivation can lead to a decrease in immune function. Lack of sleep reduces the production of protective cytokines and can diminish the activity of T cells. This weakening of the immune system makes the body more susceptible to infections and can prolong recovery time from illness.

Sleep and Chronic Inflammation

Chronic inflammation is a key factor in the aging process and the development of age-related diseases. Poor sleep quality and sleep disturbances can exacerbate inflammatory responses, contributing to the progression of diseases like heart disease, diabetes, and arthritis. By promoting better sleep, we can help mitigate chronic inflammation and its deleterious effects on the body.

The Role of Sleep in Disease Prevention

Cardiovascular Health

Good sleep is essential for maintaining cardiovascular health. Sleep affects blood pressure, heart rate, and levels of certain chemicals in the blood that can influence heart health. Disrupted sleep patterns are linked to an increased risk of hypertension, heart attacks, and strokes.

Metabolic Health

Sleep plays a significant role in maintaining metabolic health. It influences glucose metabolism and insulin sensitivity, critical factors in the prevention of type 2 diabetes. Adequate sleep helps regulate hormones that control appetite, thus playing a role in weight management and obesity prevention.

Neurological Health

Sleep is crucial for brain health. It aids in the clearance of brain waste products, including beta-amyloid, a protein associated with Alzheimer's disease. By supporting brain health through sleep, we can reduce the risk of neurodegenerative diseases.

Strategies to Enhance Sleep for Immune Health

Prioritizing Sleep

Making sleep a priority is essential for immune health. This includes setting aside enough time for sleep and creating a consistent sleep schedule.

Relaxation Techniques

Practices such as meditation, deep breathing, and gentle yoga can promote relaxation and improve sleep quality, thereby supporting the immune system.

Diet and Exercise

A balanced diet and regular exercise can enhance sleep quality. Foods rich in antioxidants and anti-inflammatory properties can support immune health, while physical activity can improve sleep efficiency and duration.

Sleep Environment

Creating a conducive sleep environment — quiet, dark, and comfortable — can significantly improve sleep quality, thus supporting the immune system.

Stress Management

Managing stress through activities like hobbies, social engagement, and relaxation practices can improve sleep quality and, in turn, boost immune function.

Conclusion

The relationship between sleep and the immune system is a critical aspect of combating aging and disease. By understanding and harnessing the power of sleep, we can significantly bolster our immune defenses, paving the way for a healthier, more resilient body as we age.

The Impact of Sleep on Heart Health, Weight Management, and Chronic Conditions

The influence of sleep extends beyond mere rest, playing a pivotal role in heart health, weight management, and the management of chronic conditions. In this book we explore how sleep intertwines with these crucial aspects of physical health, revealing the far-reaching implications of sleep on our overall well-being.

Sleep and Heart Health

The heart, a tireless worker in the human body, finds its respite and rejuvenation during sleep. Quality sleep contributes to the maintenance of cardiovascular health in several significant ways.

Regulation of Blood Pressure and Heart Rate

Sleep aids in regulating blood pressure and heart rate. During the deeper stages of sleep, the body experiences drops in blood pressure, offering a period of rest to the cardiovascular system. Consistent lack of sleep or poor sleep quality can lead to higher nighttime blood pressure, a risk factor for heart disease.

Impact on Inflammation and Stress

Sleep also plays a role in controlling inflammation and stress hormones, both of which are linked to heart health. Chronic sleep deprivation can lead to elevated levels of stress hormones like cortisol and inflammatory markers, increasing the risk of cardiovascular diseases.

Correlation with Heart Diseases

Studies have shown that individuals who experience sleep disturbances or sleep disorders such as sleep apnea are at a higher risk of developing heart diseases. Sleep apnea, characterized by repeated breathing interruptions during sleep, is associated with arrhythmias, heart attacks, and strokes.

Sleep and Weight Management

The interplay between sleep and weight management is a complex but crucial aspect of health. Sleep influences various hormones and processes that are directly related to weight management.

Hormonal Balance

Sleep affects the balance of hormones that control appetite — ghrelin and leptin. Ghrelin stimulates hunger, while leptin signals satiety to the brain. Lack of sleep can increase ghrelin levels and decrease leptin levels, leading to increased hunger and appetite, often resulting in weight gain.

Metabolism and Insulin Sensitivity

Sleep deprivation can also affect the body's metabolism and its ability to process glucose. Insufficient sleep can lead to a pre-diabetic state, reduce insulin sensitivity, and disrupt glucose metabolism, contributing to weight gain and the risk of developing type 2 diabetes.

Energy Levels and Physical Activity

Poor sleep can lead to decreased energy levels and reduced physical activity. Fatigue and lethargy can result in less motivation to engage in exercise or physical activity, further contributing to weight gain and obesity.

Sleep and Chronic Conditions

Sleep has a profound impact on various chronic conditions, influencing both their development and management.

Diabetes

For individuals with diabetes, sleep plays a critical role in managing blood sugar levels. Both quantity and quality of sleep can affect glucose metabolism and insulin sensitivity. Disrupted sleep patterns can exacerbate the symptoms of diabetes, making management more challenging.

Respiratory Diseases

Conditions like asthma and chronic obstructive pulmonary disease (COPD) can be affected by sleep quality. Poor sleep can exacerbate respiratory symptoms, while conditions like sleep apnea can further impair respiratory function.

Arthritis and Chronic Pain

Sleep and pain are closely related. Chronic pain can disrupt sleep, while poor sleep can increase the perception of pain. Good sleep hygiene and effective pain management are essential for improving sleep quality in individuals with chronic pain conditions like arthritis.

Strategies for Improving Sleep for Physical Health

Consistent Sleep Schedule

Maintaining a regular sleep schedule helps regulate the body's internal clock, improving sleep quality and duration.

Diet and Exercise

A balanced diet and regular physical activity can positively impact sleep quality. Avoiding heavy meals, caffeine, and alcohol before bedtime is crucial.

Stress Management

Managing stress through relaxation techniques, mindfulness, and recreational activities can improve sleep quality, thereby benefiting physical health.

Sleep Environment

Creating a conducive environment for sleep — cool, quiet, and comfortable — can significantly enhance sleep quality.

Medical Consultation for Sleep Disorders

Seeking medical advice for sleep disorders such as insomnia or sleep apnea is crucial. Timely diagnosis and treatment can prevent the exacerbation of chronic conditions and improve overall health.

Conclusion

Sleep's role in heart health, weight management, and chronic conditions is integral and multifaceted. By understanding and optimizing our sleep, we can positively influence these aspects of health, contributing significantly to our physical well-being.

Hormonal Balance and Sleep: Its Effect on Aging

The intricate dance between hormonal balance and sleep plays a crucial role in the aging process. Hormones, the body's chemical messengers, are significantly influenced by sleep patterns and in turn, affect various aspects of health and aging. In "Dreaming of Youth," we delve into how sleep impacts hormonal balance and the subsequent effects on the aging process.

The Interplay Between Sleep and Hormones

Sleep and hormonal systems are deeply interconnected. The quality and quantity of sleep can directly influence the secretion and regulation of various hormones, which are integral to physical and mental health.

Impact on Growth Hormone

Growth hormone, essential for cell repair and regeneration, is predominantly secreted during deep sleep stages. It plays a vital role in tissue repair, muscle growth, and bone density. Insufficient sleep can lead to decreased levels of growth hormone, potentially accelerating the aging process and diminishing the body's capacity for repair and rejuvenation.

Regulation of Stress Hormones

Cortisol, the primary stress hormone, follows a diurnal rhythm closely tied to the sleep-wake cycle. Chronic sleep deprivation can lead to prolonged elevation of cortisol levels, which in turn can have various deleterious health effects, including impaired cognitive function, decreased bone density, and a weakened immune system. This disruption can accelerate aspects of the aging process.

Sleep and Sex Hormones

Sleep also influences the production of sex hormones such as estrogen and testosterone. These hormones are essential not only for reproductive health but also for maintaining muscle mass, bone density, and overall vitality. Disrupted sleep patterns, common in aging adults, can lead to imbalances in these hormones, affecting sexual health, mood, and energy levels.

Melatonin and Aging

Melatonin, known as the sleep hormone, is critical for regulating the sleep-wake cycle. Its production decreases with age, which can contribute to sleep disturbances in older adults. Melatonin has antioxidant properties and is believed to play a role in slowing down the aging process. Its decline can thus have implications not only for sleep quality but also for the overall aging process.

The Effect of Hormonal Imbalances on Sleep

Just as sleep affects hormonal balance, hormonal imbalances can impact sleep quality.

Menopause and Sleep

During menopause, fluctuations in estrogen and progesterone can lead to sleep disturbances. Hot flashes and night sweats can disrupt sleep, while lower levels of estrogen can contribute to insomnia. These changes can affect sleep quality, impacting overall health and accelerating certain aspects of aging.

Andropause and Sleep in Men

Andropause, the male equivalent of menopause characterized by a decline in testosterone levels, can also impact sleep. Lower testosterone levels are associated with reduced sleep efficiency, less deep sleep, and increased awakenings. These changes can contribute to fatigue, mood disturbances, and a decline in physical health, influencing the aging process.

Strategies to Support Hormonal Balance Through Sleep

Prioritizing Sleep

Ensuring adequate and quality sleep is paramount in maintaining hormonal balance. Adults should aim for 7-9 hours of sleep per night, adjusting schedules and routines to accommodate this need.

Managing Light Exposure

Light exposure, particularly blue light from screens, can disrupt melatonin production. Reducing screen time before bed and exposing oneself to natural light during the day can help regulate melatonin levels.

Stress Management

Effective stress management can regulate cortisol levels. Relaxation techniques, mindfulness, and leisure activities can help mitigate stress and improve sleep quality.

Diet and Nutrition

A balanced diet rich in nutrients can support hormonal health. Certain foods can promote sleep, such as those containing tryptophan, magnesium, and calcium, while others like caffeine and sugar should be limited, especially close to bedtime.

Regular Exercise

Regular physical activity, particularly aerobic exercise, can improve sleep quality and support hormonal balance. However, it's important to avoid intense workouts close to bedtime, as they can be stimulating.

Consultation with Healthcare Providers

Regular check-ups and discussions with healthcare providers can help identify and address any hormonal imbalances. Hormone replacement therapy or other treatments should be considered under medical guidance.

Conclusion

The relationship between sleep, hormonal balance, and aging is complex and significant. By understanding and optimizing our sleep, we can positively influence hormonal balance, which in turn can slow down certain aspects of the aging process and improve overall health.

Chapter 4: Mental Health and Cognitive Function

The Connection Between Sleep, Mood, and Mental Health

In the intricate web of factors that influence our mental well-being, sleep emerges as a critical yet often overlooked thread. The connection between sleep, mood, and mental health is profound, influencing our daily lives in myriad ways. In this chapter of "Dreaming of Youth," we explore this vital relationship and how understanding it can pave the way to better mental health and cognitive function.

The Bidirectional Relationship Between Sleep and Mental Health

The relationship between sleep and mental health is inherently bidirectional. On one hand, poor sleep can be a precursor to mental health issues; on the other, existing mental health conditions can exacerbate sleep problems. This cyclical nature makes understanding and addressing sleep issues an essential component of mental health care.

Sleep's Impact on Mood

One of the most immediate effects of inadequate sleep is its impact on mood. Lack of sleep can lead to irritability, short temper, and vulnerability to stress. Chronic sleep deprivation is associated with higher rates of mood disorders, anxiety, and depression. Sleep affects neurotransmitter and stress hormone levels, both of which play a crucial role in mood regulation.

The Role of REM Sleep in Emotional Processing

REM sleep, the stage associated with vivid dreaming, is particularly important for emotional regulation. During REM sleep, the brain processes emotional experiences and helps regulate the emotional tone. This stage of sleep contributes to our ability to cope with stress and manage emotional challenges.

Sleep Disorders and Mental Health Conditions

Sleep disorders such as insomnia and sleep apnea are not just disturbances of sleep; they are often intertwined with mental health conditions.

Insomnia and Mental Health

Insomnia, characterized by difficulty falling or staying asleep, is commonly linked with depression and anxiety disorders. It can precede the onset of these conditions or exacerbate existing symptoms. Addressing insomnia can often lead to improvements in mental health.

Sleep Apnea and Its Psychological Impact

Sleep apnea, a condition marked by interrupted breathing during sleep, can lead to fragmented sleep and reduced oxygen levels in the blood. These disturbances can have significant psychological effects, including increased risk for depression, anxiety, and cognitive impairment.

The Impact of Sleep on Cognitive Functions

The quality and quantity of sleep also have direct implications for cognitive functions such as memory, concentration, and decision-making.

Memory Consolidation

Sleep plays a crucial role in memory consolidation. During sleep, especially during deep and REM stages, the brain processes and consolidates memories from the day. Poor sleep can impair this process, leading to difficulties in learning and memory retention.

Concentration and Decision-Making

Adequate sleep is essential for optimal brain function. Lack of sleep can impair attention, alertness, and the ability to solve problems. This can affect everyday decision-making, from minor choices to significant life decisions.

Strategies to Improve Sleep for Better Mental Health

To harness the benefits of good sleep for mental health, several strategies can be employed:

Establishing a Regular Sleep Routine

A consistent sleep schedule helps regulate the body's internal clock, improving sleep quality and mood. This includes going to bed and waking up at the same time every day.

Creating a Sleep-Inducing Environment

A comfortable, quiet, and dark sleeping environment can enhance the quality of sleep. This may involve investing in comfortable bedding, using blackout curtains, and maintaining an ideal room temperature.

Mindfulness and Relaxation Techniques

Practices like meditation, deep breathing, or progressive muscle relaxation can be effective in promoting relaxation and easing the transition to sleep.

Limiting Screen Time

Reducing exposure to screens and blue light, especially before bedtime, can improve sleep quality. Blue light can suppress the production of melatonin, a hormone that regulates sleep.

Physical Activity

Regular physical activity, particularly aerobic exercises, can improve sleep quality and mood. However, it's advisable to avoid intense workouts close to bedtime.

Seeking Professional Help

For persistent sleep problems or mental health issues, seeking help from a healthcare professional is important. They can provide tailored advice, therapy options, or medication if needed.

Conclusion

The interplay between sleep, mood, and mental health is a vital aspect of our overall well-being. By understanding and addressing our sleep needs, we can significantly impact our mental health, mood, and cognitive abilities.

Sleep and Cognitive Abilities: Memory, Focus, and Creativity

The role of sleep in shaping our cognitive abilities is profound and multifaceted. From memory consolidation to enhancing focus and sparking creativity, sleep is an indispensable ally in our cognitive function. In this chapter of "Dreaming of Youth," we dive into the fascinating relationship between sleep and the triumvirate of cognitive powers: memory, focus, and creativity.

Sleep's Influence on Memory

One of the most critical cognitive functions impacted by sleep is memory. Sleep plays a key role in both the consolidation and retrieval of memories.

Memory Consolidation During Sleep

Sleep is crucial for memory consolidation — the process of converting short-term memories into long-term ones. This occurs predominantly during the deep and REM stages of sleep, when the brain replays the day's events, strengthening neural connections. This process not only helps in embedding memories but also in making them more accessible for future retrieval.

The Different Types of Memory Affected

Both declarative memory (facts and information) and procedural memory (skills and tasks) benefit from good sleep. For instance, students who get adequate sleep after studying tend to perform better on tests, indicating enhanced memory consolidation.

The Role of Sleep in Focus and Concentration

Adequate sleep is essential for maintaining focus and concentration — abilities that are crucial for learning, problem-solving, and daily functioning.

Sleep Deprivation and Attention

Lack of sleep can significantly impair attention and the ability to focus. Even partial sleep deprivation can lead to reduced alertness and a shortened attention span, impacting both academic performance and day-to-day tasks.

The Impact on Cognitive Overload

A well-rested brain is better equipped to handle cognitive overload — the bombardment of information and stimuli we often face in our modern, fast-paced world. Sleep helps in "resetting" the brain, allowing for better focus and concentration the following day.

Sleep and Creativity

Sleep is also a vital ingredient in the recipe for creativity. It influences creative thinking and the ability to come up with innovative solutions.

The Connection Between REM Sleep and Creativity

REM sleep, in particular, has been linked with creative problem-solving. The free-flowing thoughts and lack of linear thinking during dreaming can lead to novel connections and ideas. Artists, writers, and inventors often attribute sleep as a source of creative inspiration.

Integrating New Knowledge

Sleep not only helps in solidifying what we have learned but also in integrating new knowledge with existing information. This integration is essential for creativity, as it allows for the combination of different ideas and concepts to form new, creative thoughts.

Strategies to Enhance Cognitive Abilities Through Sleep

To maximize the cognitive benefits of sleep, certain strategies can be adopted:

Prioritizing Quality Sleep

Ensuring you get enough high-quality sleep is crucial. This means aiming for 7-9 hours of uninterrupted sleep and focusing on improving sleep quality, not just duration.

Establishing a Sleep-Inducing Routine

Developing a calming bedtime routine can signal to your body that it's time to wind down. This may include reading, taking a warm bath, or practicing relaxation techniques.

Creating an Optimal Sleep Environment

A comfortable, quiet, and dark environment can significantly enhance sleep quality. Investing in a good mattress and pillows, using blackout curtains, and maintaining a cool room temperature can all contribute to better sleep.

Mindful of Diet and Exercise

Diet and exercise play a significant role in sleep quality. Avoiding caffeine and heavy meals before bedtime can improve sleep, while regular exercise, particularly aerobic activities, can enhance both sleep quality and cognitive function.

Managing Stress

High stress levels can impede the ability to fall asleep and negatively impact cognitive functions. Engaging in stress-reducing activities and practicing mindfulness can help in managing stress levels, leading to better sleep and improved cognitive abilities.

Conclusion

The profound impact of sleep on cognitive abilities such as memory, focus, and creativity is undeniable. By understanding and nurturing our sleep, we can significantly enhance these cognitive functions, leading to better performance in our daily tasks and a more fulfilling intellectual life.

Preventing Age-Related Cognitive Decline Through Sleep

In the quest to maintain cognitive sharpness as we age, the role of sleep emerges as a vital yet often underestimated factor. Cognitive decline, a concern for many as they enter their later years, can be influenced significantly by sleep patterns and habits. In "Dreaming of Youth," we delve into how prioritizing sleep can be a key strategy in preventing age-related cognitive decline.

Understanding the Link Between Sleep and Cognitive Health

The connection between sleep and cognitive health is complex and profound. Quality sleep is not only essential for daily cognitive function but also plays a long-term role in maintaining cognitive health as we age.

Sleep and Brain Health

During sleep, the brain engages in critical processes such as memory consolidation and the removal of toxins and waste products. One such waste product is beta-amyloid, a protein associated with Alzheimer's disease. Adequate sleep helps in clearing beta-amyloid, potentially reducing the risk of developing neurodegenerative diseases.

The Impact of Sleep Disorders

Sleep disorders, such as insomnia and sleep apnea, can have a detrimental impact on cognitive health. Chronic sleep disturbances are linked to an increased risk of cognitive decline and dementia. Addressing these disorders can be a crucial step in maintaining cognitive health.

The Role of Sleep in Memory and Learning

Memory and learning are deeply intertwined with sleep. Sleep supports various types of memory, including declarative (facts and information) and procedural (skills and tasks).

Memory Consolidation During Sleep

Sleep facilitates the consolidation of memories, a process where short-term memories are transformed into long-term ones. This occurs mainly during deep and REM sleep stages, making uninterrupted sleep crucial for memory retention.

Learning and Neuroplasticity

Sleep also supports neuroplasticity — the brain's ability to reorganize and form new neural connections. This ability is essential for learning new information and adapting to changes, underscoring the importance of sleep in lifelong learning and cognitive agility.

Sleep's Impact on Focus and Attention

As we age, maintaining focus and attention can become more challenging. Sleep plays a significant role in these cognitive faculties.

Enhancing Concentration

Adequate sleep enhances the brain's ability to concentrate and maintain attention, critical for effective problem-solving and decision-making.

Counteracting the Effects of Aging on Attention

While aging can affect the brain's attentional capacities, regular, quality sleep can help counteract these effects, supporting sustained cognitive performance.

Strategies for Promoting Cognitive Health Through Sleep

Prioritizing Sleep Hygiene

Good sleep hygiene is essential for quality sleep. This includes maintaining a consistent sleep schedule, ensuring a comfortable sleep environment, and avoiding stimulants like caffeine and nicotine before bedtime.

Addressing Sleep Disorders

It's important to seek medical advice for sleep disorders such as insomnia or sleep apnea. Effective treatment can significantly improve sleep quality and cognitive health.

Cognitive Activities Before Bed

Engaging in cognitive activities such as reading or puzzles before bed can be beneficial, but it's important to balance this with relaxation to ensure easy transition to sleep.

Physical Activity and Diet

Regular physical activity and a balanced diet can improve sleep quality and cognitive function. Exercise promotes better sleep and reduces the risk of sleep disorders, while a nutritious diet supports overall brain health.

Stress Management

Managing stress through relaxation techniques, mindfulness, and hobbies can improve sleep quality, thereby supporting cognitive health.

Conclusion

Prioritizing sleep is a crucial, yet often overlooked, strategy in preventing age-related cognitive decline. By understanding the link between sleep and cognitive health, and implementing strategies to improve sleep quality, we can support our cognitive abilities as we age.

Chapter 5:
Sleep Disorders and Their Impact on Aging

Common Sleep Disorders and Their Effects on Health and Longevity

The realm of sleep disorders is vast, encompassing various conditions that can significantly impact health and longevity. Understanding these disorders is crucial, as they often go unrecognized or untreated, leading to long-term health consequences. In "Dreaming of Youth," we explore common sleep disorders and their potential impact on overall health and longevity.

Insomnia: More Than Just Sleeplessness

Insomnia, characterized by difficulty falling asleep, staying asleep, or both, is one of the most common sleep disorders. Its effects extend far beyond mere tiredness.

Impact on Mental Health

Chronic insomnia is strongly linked to mental health issues such as depression, anxiety, and stress-related disorders. The constant struggle to achieve restful sleep can lead to a cycle of anxiety and worry about sleep, exacerbating the condition.

Physical Health Risks

Insomnia also poses risks to physical health. It is associated with increased risks of hypertension, heart disease, and type 2 diabetes. The persistent lack of restorative sleep can lead to systemic inflammation and hormonal imbalances, contributing to these conditions.

Sleep Apnea: The Silent Disruptor

Sleep apnea, particularly obstructive sleep apnea (OSA), is a condition marked by repeated interruptions in breathing during sleep. These interruptions can have far-reaching health implications.

Cardiovascular Strain

OSA is closely linked to cardiovascular problems. The repeated episodes of low oxygen levels during sleep put a strain on the heart, increasing the risk of hypertension, heart attack, stroke, and irregular heart rhythms.

Metabolic Impact

Sleep apnea can also impact metabolic health. The disorder is associated with insulin resistance and a higher risk of developing type 2 diabetes. The disruption of sleep architecture affects the body's ability to regulate glucose effectively.

Restless Legs Syndrome: Discomfort and Disruption

Restless Legs Syndrome (RLS) is a neurological disorder characterized by an irresistible urge to move the legs, often accompanied by uncomfortable sensations. The symptoms typically worsen during rest or at night.

Sleep Quality Deterioration

RLS can severely impact sleep quality. The discomfort and need to move can lead to frequent awakenings and a reduction in deep sleep stages, leading to daytime fatigue and reduced alertness.

Mental Health Consequences

The chronic discomfort and sleep disturbances associated with RLS can lead to mood disturbances and a decreased quality of life. The condition is often associated with stress, anxiety, and depression.

Narcolepsy: The Challenge of Staying Awake

Narcolepsy is a chronic neurological disorder characterized by excessive daytime sleepiness and sudden attacks of sleep. It can profoundly affect daily life.

Disrupted Daily Functioning

Individuals with narcolepsy often struggle with maintaining regular activities due to sudden sleep attacks. This can affect work, driving, and social interactions, impacting the overall quality of life.

Sleep Architecture Disruption

Narcolepsy affects the normal sleep architecture, leading to fragmented nighttime sleep and rapid entry into REM sleep. This can result in poor sleep quality and a lack of restorative sleep.

Strategies for Managing Sleep Disorders

To mitigate the impact of sleep disorders on health and longevity, several strategies can be employed:

Professional Diagnosis and Treatment

Seeking a professional diagnosis is crucial for effective treatment. Treatments may include lifestyle changes, medications, or in the case of sleep apnea, devices like CPAP machines.

Sleep Hygiene Practices

Good sleep hygiene can alleviate some symptoms of sleep disorders. This includes maintaining a regular sleep schedule, creating a comfortable sleep environment, and avoiding stimulants before bedtime.

Cognitive Behavioral Therapy

For conditions like insomnia, cognitive behavioral therapy for insomnia (CBT-I) can be highly effective. This therapy addresses the thoughts and behaviors that contribute to insomnia.

Lifestyle Modifications

Lifestyle changes such as weight management, quitting smoking, and reducing alcohol intake can be beneficial, particularly for conditions like sleep apnea.

Conclusion

Recognizing and addressing common sleep disorders is crucial for maintaining health and prolonging longevity. These conditions, if left untreated, can lead to serious health complications and diminish the quality of life.

Strategies and Treatments for Managing Sleep Disorders

Sleep disorders, ranging from insomnia to sleep apnea, can profoundly impact health and quality of life, especially as we age. Effectively managing these disorders is crucial for maintaining overall well-being and longevity. In "Dreaming of Youth," we delve into various strategies and treatments that can aid in managing sleep disorders, helping individuals achieve restful and restorative sleep.

Understanding Sleep Disorders

Before delving into management strategies, it's essential to understand the nature of the sleep disorder. Each condition, whether it's insomnia, sleep apnea, restless legs syndrome, or narcolepsy, requires a tailored approach. Diagnosis by a healthcare professional is key to determining the specific type and cause of the sleep disorder.

Insomnia: Addressing the Mind and Environment

Insomnia, characterized by difficulty falling or staying asleep, can often be managed through lifestyle changes and cognitive-behavioral approaches.

Cognitive Behavioral Therapy for Insomnia (CBT-I)

CBT-I is a highly effective treatment for insomnia. It involves changing the thoughts and behaviors that disrupt sleep, developing better sleep habits, and reducing anxiety about sleep.

Sleep Hygiene

Improving sleep hygiene can have a significant impact. This includes establishing a consistent sleep schedule, creating a conducive sleep environment, and avoiding caffeine, nicotine, and alcohol before bed.

Sleep Apnea: From Lifestyle Changes to Medical Devices

Obstructive sleep apnea (OSA) requires specific interventions to ensure uninterrupted breathing during sleep.

Continuous Positive Airway Pressure (CPAP) Therapy

CPAP therapy is the most common treatment for moderate to severe sleep apnea. It involves wearing a mask that delivers a constant stream of air, keeping the airways open during sleep.

Lifestyle Modifications

Weight loss, if overweight, can significantly improve or even eliminate sleep apnea symptoms. Avoiding alcohol and sleeping pills, which can relax the throat muscles, is also beneficial.

Restless Legs Syndrome (RLS): Combating Discomfort

RLS, a neurological disorder that causes an irresistible urge to move the legs, can disrupt sleep. Managing it involves both lifestyle interventions and possibly medication.

Iron Supplementation

RLS is often linked to low iron levels in the brain. Iron supplements, under a doctor's supervision, can alleviate symptoms.

Medications

Medications, such as those used to treat Parkinson's disease, seizures, or neuropathy, can be effective in reducing the symptoms of RLS.

Narcolepsy: Managing Daytime Sleepiness

Narcolepsy, characterized by excessive daytime sleepiness and sudden bouts of sleep, can be managed through medications and lifestyle adjustments.

Medications

Stimulant medications can help manage the excessive daytime sleepiness, while other medications can help control cataplexy and other symptoms of narcolepsy.

Scheduled Naps

Taking short, scheduled naps at strategic times can significantly reduce sleepiness and improve alertness.

General Strategies for Managing Sleep Disorders

Beyond specific treatments, there are general strategies beneficial for various sleep disorders.

Regular Physical Activity

Regular exercise can improve sleep quality and duration. However, it's best to avoid vigorous workouts close to bedtime, as they can be too stimulating.

Mindfulness and Relaxation Techniques

Practices such as meditation, yoga, and deep breathing exercises can reduce stress and promote better sleep.

Monitoring and Adjusting Medications

Some medications can interfere with sleep. Consulting with a healthcare provider to review current medications and their impact on sleep is important.

Support and Education

Joining a support group or seeking educational resources can provide valuable tips and emotional support for managing sleep disorders.

Conclusion

Managing sleep disorders is a multifaceted process that often involves a combination of lifestyle changes, behavioral therapies, and medical treatments. Understanding the specific disorder and working closely with healthcare professionals are key to developing an effective management plan. By addressing these disorders, individuals can significantly improve their sleep quality, thereby enhancing their overall health and well-being.

Case Studies: Real-Life Impacts of Improved Sleep on Healthspan

The journey to understand and appreciate the profound impact of sleep on health and longevity can be illuminated through real-life case studies. These stories not only humanize the science behind sleep but also offer valuable insights into how improving sleep can enhance one's healthspan. In "Dreaming of Youth," we explore several case studies that highlight the transformative power of prioritizing sleep.

Case Study 1: The Corporate Executive with Insomnia

Background

John, a 52-year-old corporate executive, struggled with insomnia for years. His high-stress job and irregular travel schedule contributed to erratic sleep patterns, leading to chronic sleep deprivation.

The Intervention

John's journey to better sleep began with a consultation with a sleep specialist, who recommended Cognitive Behavioral Therapy for Insomnia (CBT-I). He also adopted a consistent sleep schedule and improved his sleep hygiene by limiting screen time before bed and creating a relaxing bedtime routine.

The Outcome

Over several months, John experienced a remarkable improvement in his sleep quality. This change led to enhanced concentration and productivity at work. His mood improved, and he reported feeling more energetic and less irritable. Remarkably, his annual health check-up showed improved markers for heart health and reduced risk factors for diabetes.

Case Study 2: The Retiree with Sleep Apnea

Background

Margaret, a 65-year-old retiree, had been suffering from unexplained fatigue and mood swings. A sleep study revealed moderate obstructive sleep apnea (OSA).

The Intervention

Margaret was prescribed Continuous Positive Airway Pressure (CPAP) therapy. Initially resistant to using the CPAP machine, she eventually adapted to it with support from her healthcare provider and a local support group.

The Outcome

With consistent use of the CPAP machine, Margaret's sleep quality drastically improved. She experienced fewer daytime naps, her energy levels increased, and her mood stabilized. She also noticed an improvement in her cognitive functions, such as memory and concentration.

Case Study 3: The College Student with Delayed Sleep Phase Syndrome

Background

Alex, a 20-year-old college student, had a lifelong habit of going to bed late and struggling to wake up for morning classes, indicative of Delayed Sleep Phase Syndrome.

The Intervention

Alex underwent light therapy, using a light box upon waking to help reset his circadian rhythm. He also adopted a more regular sleep schedule, avoiding caffeine in the evening and engaging in relaxing activities before bedtime.

The Outcome

Alex's sleep patterns normalized over several months. He reported feeling more alert and attentive during his morning classes, and his academic performance improved. He also experienced less anxiety and better overall mood.

Case Study 4: The Middle-Aged Woman with Restless Legs Syndrome

Background

Lisa, a 45-year-old woman, experienced uncomfortable sensations in her legs at night, leading to disrupted sleep and daytime fatigue, classic symptoms of Restless Legs Syndrome (RLS).

The Intervention

After consulting with her doctor, Lisa started on iron supplements and a medication typically used for neuropathic pain. She also incorporated gentle evening exercises and warm baths into her routine.

The Outcome

The combined approach significantly reduced her RLS symptoms. Lisa started to enjoy more restful nights and her overall energy levels during the day improved. She also reported a decrease in stress and anxiety.

The Common Thread: Holistic Approach and Improved Healthspan

These case studies share a common theme: a holistic approach to managing sleep disorders can lead to significant improvements in healthspan. Each individual, by addressing their unique sleep issues, experienced not just better sleep, but also improvements in their physical, cognitive, and emotional well-being.

Conclusion

These real-life stories underscore the critical role of sleep in enhancing health and longevity. They demonstrate that with the right interventions and commitment, it is possible to overcome sleep challenges and significantly improve one's quality of life.

Chapter 6: Enhancing Sleep Quality

Practical Tips for Improving Sleep Hygiene

In the pursuit of better sleep, the concept of sleep hygiene plays a pivotal role. Sleep hygiene involves practices and habits that are conducive to sleeping well on a regular basis. In "Dreaming of Youth," we explore practical tips to enhance sleep hygiene, offering a pathway to improved sleep quality and, consequently, a healthier life.

Understanding the Importance of Sleep Hygiene

Good sleep hygiene is essential for high-quality sleep, which is crucial for overall health and well-being. It's about creating an environment and adopting habits that foster uninterrupted and restful sleep. Poor sleep hygiene can lead to sleep disturbances, insomnia, and can exacerbate other sleep disorders.

Establishing a Consistent Sleep Schedule

One of the foundational aspects of good sleep hygiene is maintaining a regular sleep schedule. Going to bed and waking up at the same time every day, including weekends, helps regulate the body's internal clock and can improve sleep quality over time. Consistency is key in aligning our natural circadian rhythms with our daily routines.

Creating a Conducive Sleep Environment

The environment in which we sleep can have a profound impact on the quality of our rest. The bedroom should be a sanctuary designed for sleep.

Comfortable Bedding

Investing in a comfortable mattress and pillows can make a significant difference. The preferences for mattress firmness and pillow type can vary, so it's important to choose what feels most comfortable.

Room Temperature

The temperature of the room can greatly affect sleep quality. Most people sleep best in a slightly cool room, around 65 degrees Fahrenheit (18 degrees Celsius).

Reducing Light and Noise

Excessive light and noise can disrupt sleep. Using blackout curtains and considering earplugs or white noise machines can help create a more serene sleeping environment.

Monitoring Diet and Fluid Intake

What we eat and drink before bed can influence our sleep. A heavy meal or spicy foods can cause discomfort and indigestion, disrupting sleep. It's advisable to eat dinner at least a few hours before bedtime. Limiting fluid intake before bed can reduce nighttime trips to the bathroom.

Caffeine and Alcohol

Caffeine and alcohol can also interfere with sleep. Avoiding caffeine in the afternoon and evening and minimizing alcohol consumption can promote better sleep quality.

Establishing a Pre-Sleep Routine

A relaxing pre-sleep routine can signal to your body that it's time to wind down. This might include activities like reading, taking a warm bath, or practicing relaxation techniques such as deep breathing or gentle stretching. The key is to find activities that are calming and make them a regular part of the bedtime routine.

Managing Screen Time

In our digital age, screens are a significant part of our lives, but their use before bedtime can be detrimental to sleep. The blue light emitted by screens can suppress the production of melatonin, the hormone that controls sleep-wake cycles. Limiting screen use an hour before bed can help avoid this issue.

Physical Activity

Regular physical activity can improve sleep quality, especially aerobic exercises like walking, swimming, or cycling. However, timing is important; engaging in vigorous exercise too close to bedtime can be stimulating and may hinder the ability to fall asleep.

Dealing with Stress

Stress and sleep have a complex relationship. High stress levels can make it difficult to fall asleep and stay asleep. Finding effective ways to manage stress — such as mindfulness meditation, yoga, or journaling — can improve sleep quality.

Being Wary of Sleep Aids

While over-the-counter and prescription sleep aids can be helpful in the short term, they are not a long-term solution and can sometimes lead to dependency or tolerance. It's important to use them cautiously and under the guidance of a healthcare provider.

Seeking Professional Help When Necessary

If sleep disturbances persist despite good sleep hygiene practices, it may be necessary to seek professional help. A healthcare provider can offer guidance and treatment options, including referrals to a sleep specialist if needed.

Conclusion

Improving sleep hygiene is a crucial step towards achieving better sleep and, by extension, a healthier, more energetic life. By adopting these practical tips, individuals can create an environment and habits conducive to restful sleep, laying the foundation for improved health and well-being.

The Role of Diet, Exercise, and Lifestyle in Sleep Quality

The quest for better sleep is not just confined to the bedroom; it extends to our plates, our physical activities, and our daily routines. The quality of sleep we enjoy is intricately linked with our diet, exercise habits, and overall lifestyle. In "Dreaming of Youth," we delve into how these elements collectively influence sleep quality, offering a holistic approach to enhancing sleep.

The Interplay Between Diet and Sleep

What we eat and when we eat plays a pivotal role in how well we sleep. Our dietary choices can either promote restful sleep or contribute to sleep disturbances.

Nutritional Balance and Sleep

A balanced diet rich in fruits, vegetables, whole grains, and lean proteins can have a positive impact on sleep. These foods provide essential nutrients that support the body's natural sleep processes. For example, magnesium and potassium, found in bananas and leafy greens, can help relax muscles and calm the nervous system.

Timing of Meals

Eating habits, particularly the timing of meals, can also affect sleep quality. Eating a heavy meal right before bed can lead to discomfort and indigestion, making it harder to fall asleep. Conversely, going to bed hungry can also be disruptive. The key is to find a balance, eating a light snack if needed before bedtime.

Impact of Caffeine and Alcohol

Caffeine and alcohol are two substances that can significantly impair sleep quality. Caffeine, a stimulant, can disrupt sleep patterns if consumed too late in the day. Alcohol, while initially sedative, can lead to fragmented and non-restorative sleep. Limiting caffeine intake in the afternoon and evening and moderating alcohol consumption can improve sleep quality.

The Role of Exercise in Enhancing Sleep

Regular physical activity is another crucial factor in the sleep equation. Exercise not only helps tire the body physically, promoting sleepiness, but it also has several other sleep-related benefits.

Exercise and Sleep-Wake Cycle

Physical activity, especially aerobic exercise, can help regulate the sleep-wake cycle by raising body temperature and then allowing it to drop and trigger sleepiness a few hours later. This can be particularly beneficial for those with insomnia.

Stress Reduction and Sleep

Exercise is an effective stress reliever. By reducing stress and anxiety levels, it can make it easier to fall asleep and enjoy more restful sleep.

Timing Matters

The timing of exercise can influence its impact on sleep. While morning or afternoon exercise can improve sleep quality, engaging in high-intensity workouts too close to bedtime might be overly stimulating for some people.

Lifestyle Factors Influencing Sleep Quality

Beyond diet and exercise, various lifestyle factors can either enhance or impede sleep quality. These include our daily routines, stress management practices, and even our social interactions.

The Importance of a Regular Routine

Maintaining a regular daily routine, including consistent wake-up and bedtimes, can help regulate the body's internal clock and improve sleep quality. This regularity provides a sense of rhythm and predictability that is conducive to sleep.

Stress Management Techniques

High levels of stress and worry can significantly impair the ability to fall and stay asleep. Engaging in stress management techniques like mindfulness meditation, deep breathing exercises, and yoga can help calm the mind and prepare the body for sleep.

Social and Environmental Factors

Social interactions and environmental conditions also play a role. Positive social interactions can improve mood and reduce stress, benefiting sleep. Conversely, a noisy or disruptive environment can impair sleep quality, highlighting the importance of creating a tranquil and comfortable sleep space.

Integrating Diet, Exercise, and Lifestyle for Better Sleep

To optimize sleep quality, a holistic approach that integrates diet, exercise, and lifestyle adjustments is essential.

Balancing Diet for Sleep

This means not only choosing sleep-promoting foods but also being mindful of meal timing and portion sizes. Small dietary adjustments, like reducing sugar and processed foods, especially close to bedtime, can have a significant impact.

Incorporating Regular Exercise

Incorporating physical activity into daily life, whether it's a brisk walk, a swim, or a yoga session, can enhance sleep quality. Finding an exercise routine that is enjoyable and sustainable is key.

Adapting Lifestyle Choices

Making small changes in daily routines, such as reducing screen time before bed, creating a bedtime ritual, and managing stress, can collectively improve sleep quality.

Conclusion

The journey to better sleep is multifaceted, involving more than just bedtime habits. It encompasses a balanced diet, regular exercise, and positive lifestyle choices. By understanding and incorporating these elements, we can significantly enhance our sleep quality, contributing to better health and well-being.

Alternative Therapies and Their Effectiveness: Meditation, Supplements, and More

In the pursuit of enhanced sleep quality, many turn to alternative therapies. These therapies, ranging from meditation to dietary supplements, offer diverse approaches to improving sleep. In "Dreaming of Youth," we examine various alternative therapies and assess their effectiveness in enhancing sleep quality.

Meditation and Mindfulness

Meditation and mindfulness have gained popularity as effective tools for improving sleep. Their role in stress reduction and relaxation is well-documented, making them valuable in addressing sleep issues.

Meditation and Sleep

Meditation practices, especially those focusing on relaxation and breathing, can help prepare the body and mind for sleep. By calming the mind and reducing the whirlwind of thoughts, meditation can ease the transition into sleep.

Mindfulness for Better Sleep

Mindfulness, the practice of being present and fully engaged in the current moment, can reduce bedtime anxiety and stress, common culprits of sleep disturbances. Mindfulness-based therapy for insomnia (MBTI) is a structured program that combines mindfulness meditation and behavioral changes to improve sleep.

Dietary Supplements

Various supplements are touted for their sleep-inducing properties. It's important to approach these with caution and preferably under medical supervision.

Melatonin

Melatonin supplements are commonly used to treat sleep disorders, particularly for issues like jet lag and shift work sleep disorder. As a natural hormone that regulates the sleep-wake cycle, supplemental melatonin can help realign the body's internal clock.

Herbal Supplements

Herbs like valerian root, chamomile, and lavender are known for their sedative effects. While some find these herbs helpful in promoting sleep, scientific evidence regarding their effectiveness is mixed.

Magnesium and Other Minerals

Supplements like magnesium, which plays a role in muscle relaxation and nervous system regulation, can potentially improve sleep quality. However, it's important to consult with a healthcare provider before starting any supplement regimen.

Acupuncture

Acupuncture, a traditional Chinese medicine practice, involves inserting thin needles into specific points on the body. It's thought to stimulate the nervous system and can be used to address sleep disturbances.

Acupuncture for Insomnia

Some studies suggest that acupuncture can be effective in treating insomnia. It is believed to work by inducing relaxation and modulating the production of neurotransmitters associated with sleep.

Aromatherapy

Aromatherapy uses essential oils to promote health and well-being, with certain oils reputed to encourage relaxation and sleep.

Essential Oils for Sleep

Lavender oil is widely recognized for its calming properties and is often used to improve sleep quality. Other oils like chamomile and bergamot may also be beneficial. These can be used in diffusers or applied topically in diluted form.

Yoga and Tai Chi

Gentle physical practices like yoga and tai chi can be effective in promoting relaxation and improving sleep.

Yoga's Relaxation Effects

Yoga, particularly styles that focus on slow movements and deep breathing, can be a helpful pre-sleep routine. It aids in reducing stress and calming the mind.

Tai Chi for Better Sleep

Tai Chi, a form of gentle martial arts, is known for its meditative movements. Practicing Tai Chi can reduce stress and anxiety, potentially improving sleep quality.

Sound Therapy

Sound therapy, including white noise machines or nature soundtracks, can create a soothing environment conducive to sleep.

White Noise and Sleep

White noise machines emit a consistent, ambient sound that can mask other disruptive noises. This can be particularly useful in noisy environments or for those with sensitive hearing.

Cognitive Behavioral Techniques

Cognitive behavioral techniques, though not strictly an alternative therapy, are worth mentioning for their effectiveness in improving sleep.

CBT for Insomnia

Cognitive Behavioral Therapy for Insomnia (CBT-I) is a structured program that addresses the thoughts and behaviors that disrupt sleep. It's considered one of the most effective treatments for insomnia.

Conclusion

Alternative therapies offer a range of options for those seeking to improve their sleep quality. While their effectiveness can vary from person to person, they provide valuable tools that can be incorporated into a comprehensive approach to sleep improvement. It's important to approach these therapies mindfully and, in some cases, with medical guidance.

Chapter 7: Technological Advances in Sleep Science

Wearables and Apps for Sleep Tracking and Improvement

In an era where technology intersects with almost every aspect of life, sleep science has also embraced technological advancements. Wearables and apps designed for sleep tracking and improvement have become increasingly popular, offering users insights into their sleep patterns and ways to enhance sleep quality. In "Dreaming of Youth," we explore the burgeoning world of sleep technology and its role in promoting better sleep.

The Rise of Sleep Tracking Technology

Sleep tracking technology has evolved rapidly, moving from basic pedometers to sophisticated devices that monitor various aspects of sleep. These technologies include wearable devices like smart-watches and fitness trackers, as well as smartphone apps designed to analyze sleep.

Understanding Sleep Through Data

These devices and apps typically use motion sensors and heart rate monitors to estimate sleep stages, including light, deep, and REM sleep. They provide data on sleep duration, interruptions, and sometimes even insights into breathing patterns and heart rate variability.

Wearables: More Than Just Step Counters

Wearable devices have become popular tools for sleep tracking. They offer the convenience of collecting data passively while the user sleeps.

Accuracy and Reliability

While not as accurate as clinical sleep studies, many wearables provide a reasonable estimation of sleep patterns and quality. They can be particularly useful for noticing trends over time, such as changes in sleep duration or the regularity of sleep schedules.

Features and Feedback

Many wearables come with features that offer feedback on sleep quality and provide tips for improvement. Some even include smart alarms designed to wake the user during lighter stages of sleep, potentially reducing grogginess.

Smartphone Apps for Sleep Analysis

Smartphone apps for sleep tracking have gained popularity due to their ease of use and accessibility. These apps often use the phone's accelerometer to track movement during sleep, estimating sleep cycles and quality.

App-Based Sleep Improvement Programs

Beyond tracking, some apps offer structured programs to improve sleep. These may include guided meditations, relaxation exercises, or cognitive behavioral therapy techniques.

Limitations and Privacy Concerns

It's important to note the limitations of app-based tracking, which may not be as accurate as wearable devices. Additionally, privacy concerns regarding the handling of personal sleep data should be considered.

Integrating Technology with Good Sleep Practices

While technology can provide valuable insights, it's crucial to integrate it with good sleep practices and, if necessary, professional medical advice.

Technology as a Tool, Not a Solution

Sleep tracking technology is best used as a tool to gain insights, rather than a standalone solution for sleep issues. It should complement, not replace, traditional approaches to improving sleep quality.

Avoiding Obsession with Sleep Data

There's a risk of becoming overly focused on sleep data, potentially leading to anxiety and worsened sleep. It's important to use the data constructively and not let it become a source of stress.

The Future of Sleep Technology

The future of sleep technology looks promising, with advancements in artificial intelligence and machine learning offering even more sophisticated analysis and personalized recommendations.

Predictive Analytics and Personalized Advice

Emerging technologies may be able to predict sleep disturbances before they happen and offer personalized advice to prevent them. This could lead to more proactive and effective management of sleep quality.

Integration with Health Platforms

There's potential for sleep data to be integrated into broader health platforms, providing a more holistic view of an individual's health and well-being.

Conclusion

Wearables and apps for sleep tracking represent a significant step forward in personal health technology. They offer valuable insights into our sleep patterns and provide guidance for improvement.

However, it's important to use these tools wisely, integrating them into a broader approach to sleep hygiene and consulting with healthcare professionals when necessary.

The Future of Sleep Research and Its Implications for Aging

As we continue to unravel the mysteries of sleep, the future of sleep research looks bright, with promising implications for aging and longevity. Advancements in technology, neuroscience, and genetics are opening new frontiers in our understanding of sleep and its profound impact on the aging process. Here we explore what the future may hold for sleep research and how it could transform our approach to healthy aging.

The Evolution of Sleep Science

Sleep science has come a long way from the days of simply monitoring sleep duration and disturbances. Today, it encompasses a broad range of studies from the molecular mechanisms of sleep to its impact on chronic diseases associated with aging.

Cutting-Edge Technologies in Sleep Monitoring

Emerging technologies in sleep monitoring, including wearable devices and non-invasive sensors, are becoming more sophisticated. Future devices may offer more accurate and comprehensive data on sleep stages, quality, and physiological changes during sleep.

Neuroscientific Advances

Neuroscience is delving deeper into how sleep affects brain health. Advanced imaging techniques are allowing researchers to study the brain's activity during sleep in greater detail, providing insights into how sleep contributes to cognitive functions and brain aging.

Sleep, Genetics, and Personalized Medicine

The intersection of sleep research with genetics and personalized medicine is an exciting development. Understanding the genetic basis of sleep disorders and individual sleep patterns can lead to more personalized and effective treatment approaches.

Genetic Insights into Sleep Disorders

Research into the genetic factors that influence sleep disorders may lead to targeted therapies that address the root causes of these conditions. This could be particularly beneficial for age-related sleep disorders like insomnia and sleep apnea.

Tailoring Sleep Interventions

As we understand more about the individual differences in sleep patterns and needs, sleep interventions can become more personalized. This would mean moving away from one-size-fits-all recommendations to tailored advice based on an individual's specific sleep profile.

The Link Between Sleep and Age-Related Diseases

One of the most promising areas of sleep research is its connection to age-related diseases. Understanding this link can lead to new strategies for preventing or mitigating these conditions.

Sleep and Neurodegenerative Diseases

Studies are increasingly focusing on the relationship between sleep and neurodegenerative diseases like Alzheimer's and Parkinson's. Research suggests that poor sleep may contribute to the accumulation of brain toxins and plaques associated with these diseases.

Sleep's Role in Metabolic and Cardiovascular Health

There is also growing evidence of sleep's role in metabolic and cardiovascular health. Future research may uncover more about how improving sleep can reduce the risk of conditions like diabetes and heart disease, common in older adults.

Sleep and Immune Function in Aging

The immune system and its relationship with sleep is another critical area of study, especially relevant for aging populations. As we age, our immune function naturally declines, and sleep becomes an important factor in maintaining immune health.

Enhancing Immune Resilience

Future research may reveal more about how sleep can be used to enhance immune resilience in older adults, potentially leading to strategies that boost immunity through improved sleep.

Advancements in Sleep Therapy

As research progresses, we can expect advancements in sleep therapies that go beyond treating symptoms to addressing the underlying causes of sleep disturbances.

Innovative Treatment Modalities

Emerging treatments, including light therapy, sound therapy, and even virtual reality, are being explored for their potential in improving sleep. The future may see these becoming mainstream in sleep therapy, especially for older adults.

Integration with Holistic Health Approaches

Sleep research is increasingly recognizing the importance of a holistic approach to health. This means integrating sleep therapy with other aspects of health and wellness, like diet, exercise, and mental health.

Ethical Considerations and Accessibility

As sleep research advances, it also brings forth ethical considerations and questions about accessibility. Ensuring that the benefits of advanced sleep research and technologies are available to all, regardless of socioeconomic status, is crucial.

Conclusion

The future of sleep research holds great promise for enhancing our understanding of sleep and its critical role in aging. As we continue to uncover the secrets of sleep, we can look forward to more effective interventions, personalized treatments, and a deeper understanding of how sleep can be optimized for health and longevity.

Evaluating the Effectiveness of Technological Aids in Sleep

In the modern era, technology has permeated every aspect of our lives, including our sleep. Various technological aids, from wearable devices to sleep apps and smart home systems, promise to enhance sleep quality. But how effective are these tools in reality? Here we delve into the evaluation of these technological aids, assessing their role and efficacy in improving sleep.

The Surge of Sleep Technology

The market for sleep technology has seen a significant surge, driven by a growing awareness of the importance of sleep and the appeal of easy-to-use technological solutions. These innovations range from simple apps that monitor sleep patterns to sophisticated wearables that track biometric data.

Diversity of Technological Aids

Sleep technology includes a wide array of products:

- Wearable devices like smartwatches and fitness trackers that monitor sleep stages, heart rate, and movement.

- Sleep apps that offer features like sleep tracking, meditation, and ambient sounds.

- Smart home devices such as smart mattresses and pillows, and environmental controllers that optimize bedroom conditions for sleep.

Measuring the Effectiveness of Wearables

Wearable devices have become increasingly popular for sleep tracking. They offer the convenience of passive data collection and provide insights into sleep patterns, duration, and quality.

Accuracy and Data Interpretation

While wearables offer a broad picture of sleep patterns, their accuracy, particularly in distinguishing between sleep stages, can vary. For a general understanding of sleep habits, they can be quite useful, but they are not a substitute for professional medical assessments for diagnosing sleep disorders.

Impact on Sleep Behavior

One of the key benefits of wearables is the potential to modify sleep behavior. By providing tangible data and trends, these devices can motivate individuals to adopt healthier sleep habits. However, the effectiveness largely depends on the user's engagement and willingness to implement changes based on the data provided.

The Role of Apps in Sleep Improvement

Apps designed for sleep improvement often include features like guided meditations, sleep stories, and ambient sounds. They are accessible tools for many seeking to enhance their sleep quality.

Behavioral Modification

Many sleep apps are designed to facilitate relaxation and prepare the mind for sleep. For individuals struggling with stress or an overactive mind at bedtime, these apps can be beneficial in establishing a calming pre-sleep routine.

Limitations and User Dependency

The limitations of these apps lie in their one-size-fits-all approach and the accuracy of sleep tracking using a smartphone. Additionally, there's a risk of becoming overly reliant on these apps, where the absence of the app disrupts sleep.

Smart Home Technology for Optimal Sleep Environments

Smart home technologies like intelligent lighting systems, temperature control devices, and smart mattresses can create an optimal sleep environment.

Environmental Control

Controlling environmental factors such as light, temperature, and noise can significantly improve sleep quality. Smart technology allows for personalization and automation of these aspects, potentially enhancing the sleep environment.

Personalization and Convenience

The ability to personalize and automate environmental settings based on individual preferences can make it easier to maintain consistent sleep habits. However, the effectiveness depends on correctly identifying and implementing the optimal settings for each individual.

Evaluating the Overall Impact

When evaluating the effectiveness of these technological aids, it's important to consider both the advantages and limitations.

Complementing Traditional Sleep Practices

Technology should be viewed as a complement to, not a replacement for, traditional good sleep practices. Maintaining a regular sleep schedule, practicing good sleep hygiene, and addressing any underlying sleep disorders are still fundamental.

User Engagement and Mindful Use

The efficacy of these aids depends significantly on user engagement and the mindful use of technology. Becoming overly fixated on data can lead to anxiety, counteracting the benefits. Users should aim to find a balance where technology serves as a helpful tool rather than a source of stress.

Conclusion

Technological aids for sleep, while offering valuable insights and conveniences, should be approached with a balanced perspective. Their effectiveness varies based on accuracy, personalization, and the user's approach to integrating technology with healthy sleep habits.

Chapter 8: Cultural and Societal Perspectives on Sleep

Global Sleep Patterns and Cultural Attitudes Towards Sleep

Sleep, a universal human experience, varies remarkably across different cultures and societies. These variations are not just in the duration and quality of sleep but also in the cultural attitudes and practices surrounding it. In "Dreaming of Youth," we explore the diverse tapestry of global sleep patterns and cultural attitudes, highlighting how these differences shape and reflect societal norms and values.

Understanding Global Variations in Sleep

Around the world, the way people sleep is influenced by a myriad of factors, including geography, lifestyle, societal norms, and economic conditions. These factors contribute to significant variations in sleep patterns and attitudes.

Influence of Geography and Climate

Geographical location and climate play a significant role in shaping sleep patterns. In countries near the equator, for example, the consistent length of days and nights throughout the year can influence sleep habits. In contrast, regions with extreme variations in daylight hours, like the Nordic countries, have developed different coping mechanisms and cultural practices to adapt to these environmental conditions.

Economic and Lifestyle Factors

Economic factors and lifestyle choices also significantly impact sleep. In industrialized nations, longer working hours and the prevalence of technology often lead to shorter sleep durations and later bedtimes. Conversely, in some agrarian societies, people may align their sleep schedules more closely with the natural light-dark cycle.

Cultural Attitudes Towards Sleep

Cultural attitudes towards sleep vary widely. In some cultures, sleep is regarded as a necessary but unremarkable part of the daily routine. In others, it's imbued with specific meanings and practices.

Siesta Cultures

In many parts of the world, particularly in Mediterranean and some Latin American countries, the siesta is a

cultural practice where a midday rest or nap is common. This practice, often linked to historical patterns of work and climate, shows a cultural recognition of the need for rest during the day, especially in warmer climates.

Nighttime Sleep in Western Societies

In many Western societies, there is a strong emphasis on a consolidated period of sleep during the night, typically lasting around 7-9 hours. This pattern is often dictated by the 9-to-5 work schedule and is seen as the norm for healthy sleep.

Varied Sleep Practices in Asian Cultures

In some Asian cultures, the approach to sleep can be different. For instance, in Japan, the practice of 'inemuri', or napping in public, is accepted as a sign of hard work. However, this practice exists alongside a culture of long working hours, which can lead to insufficient sleep at night.

The Impact of Technology and Globalization

The advent of technology and the influence of globalization are homogenizing sleep patterns in some respects. Exposure to screens and the internet has extended wakefulness into the night, often at the expense of sleep.

The 24/7 Society

In our increasingly connected world, the concept of a 24/7 society is emerging, where the distinction between day and night is blurred. This can lead to irregular sleep patterns and a disregard for the natural circadian rhythms that dictate sleep.

Globalization and Sleep

Globalization has also led to the spread of Western attitudes towards sleep and work, influencing sleep patterns in different cultures. The adoption of a more Westernized work schedule has led to changes in traditional sleep practices in various parts of the world.

The Importance of Understanding Cultural Differences

Recognizing and understanding these cultural differences in sleep is crucial, not only for global health initiatives but also for individuals traveling or working in different cultural contexts.

Implications for Sleep Health

Cultural attitudes towards sleep have significant implications for sleep health. Adapting sleep health interventions to fit different cultural contexts is essential for their effectiveness.

Cultural Sensitivity in Sleep Research

For sleep researchers, acknowledging and incorporating cultural variations in sleep practices is vital for a more comprehensive understanding of human sleep and its health implications.

Conclusion

Global sleep patterns and cultural attitudes towards sleep are diverse and complex. They reflect a blend of historical, geographical, economic, and social factors. In today's interconnected world, understanding these variations is more important than ever.

The Economic and Societal Impact of Sleep Deprivation

Sleep deprivation, an issue faced by millions globally, extends far beyond individual health concerns, casting a wide net over societal and economic aspects of life. Here we delve into the broader impact of sleep deprivation, examining how it affects economies and societies at large.

The Prevalence and Causes of Sleep Deprivation

In modern society, sleep deprivation is increasingly common, driven by factors such as longer work hours, increased screen time, and the blurring of work-life boundaries. This widespread lack of sleep has profound implications, not just for individuals but for communities and economies.

Work Culture and Lifestyle Choices

The culture of long working hours, especially prevalent in industrialized nations, often comes at the expense of sleep. Likewise, lifestyle choices, including the use of electronic devices before bed, contribute to delayed sleep onset and reduced sleep quality.

The Economic Costs of Sleep Deprivation

The consequences of sleep deprivation carry a substantial economic burden, impacting productivity, healthcare costs, and even workplace safety.

Reduced Productivity and Performance

Lack of sleep can significantly impair cognitive functions such as concentration, decision-making, and creativity. This leads to decreased productivity and performance at work, known as presenteeism, where employees are present but functioning suboptimally.

Increased Health Care Expenditure

Sleep deprivation is linked to a higher prevalence of chronic diseases like obesity, diabetes, and cardiovascular disease, leading to increased healthcare spending. The treatment of sleep-related disorders and the long-term management of associated health conditions add to this economic burden.

Workplace Accidents and Errors

Fatigue resulting from inadequate sleep can increase the risk of accidents and errors in the workplace. This is particularly evident in industries where safety is critical, such as healthcare, transportation, and manufacturing.

Societal Implications of Sleep Deprivation

Beyond economic factors, sleep deprivation has broad societal implications, affecting education, social interactions, and even public health.

Impact on Education and Learning

For students, insufficient sleep can impair learning, memory, and academic performance. This not only affects individual educational outcomes but can have long-term consequences on workforce readiness and skills development.

Social and Emotional Consequences

Chronic sleep deprivation can lead to irritability, mood disturbances, and impaired social interactions. This can strain personal relationships and lead to a decline in overall societal well-being.

Public Health Concerns

The public health implications of widespread sleep deprivation are significant. It contributes to the burden of chronic diseases and can exacerbate mental health issues, stretching already strained public health resources.

Addressing the Issue of Sleep Deprivation

Given the extensive impact of sleep deprivation, addressing this issue is crucial. This requires a multi-faceted approach involving policy changes, public awareness campaigns, and individual behavioral modifications.

Workplace Policies and Corporate Culture

Adopting workplace policies that prioritize work-life balance and allow for sufficient rest can help mitigate the issue. This includes regulating work hours, encouraging breaks, and providing flexibility for sleep needs.

Public Health Campaigns

Public health campaigns can play a vital role in raising awareness about the importance of sleep and its impact on health and well-being. Educating the public about good sleep hygiene and the risks of sleep deprivation can lead to healthier sleep practices.

Individual Responsibility and Lifestyle Changes

Ultimately, individuals also have a responsibility to prioritize their sleep. This includes adopting healthier sleep habits, creating a conducive sleep environment, and seeking medical help when necessary.

Conclusion

The impact of sleep deprivation extends far beyond tired individuals; it permeates the very fabric of societies and economies. Tackling this issue is not only about improving individual health outcomes but also about enhancing productivity, safety, and quality of life at a societal level.

Public Health Initiatives and Education About Sleep

In an age where sleep deprivation is increasingly common, public health initiatives and education about sleep have become more crucial than ever. These efforts aim to raise awareness about the importance of sleep and address the widespread issue of sleep disorders. Here we delve into the role of public health in promoting better sleep practices and the impact of educational efforts on societal sleep habits.

The Importance of Sleep in Public Health

Sleep is a fundamental aspect of health, yet it is often overlooked in public health discussions. Recognizing sleep as a key component of health can lead to better health outcomes and improved quality of life across populations.

Integrating Sleep into Health Policy

Integrating sleep education and promotion into public health policy is essential. This includes creating guidelines for healthy sleep, much like those for diet and exercise, and incorporating sleep into holistic health programs.

Addressing Sleep Disorders as a Public Health Issue

Sleep disorders, such as insomnia and sleep apnea, should be addressed as public health issues. Increasing screening and treatment accessibility can help reduce the burden of these disorders.

Public Health Campaigns on Sleep Education

Public health campaigns play a pivotal role in educating the public about the importance of sleep and the risks associated with sleep deprivation.

Raising Awareness

Campaigns can raise awareness about the health risks of poor sleep, including its links to chronic diseases, mental health issues, and decreased life expectancy.

Promoting Good Sleep Hygiene

Educational campaigns can also promote good sleep hygiene practices, such as maintaining a regular sleep schedule, creating a conducive sleep environment, and managing stress.

School-Based Sleep Education Programs

Schools are an ideal setting for sleep education, given the critical role of sleep in learning and development.

Incorporating Sleep Education into School Curricula

Integrating sleep education into school curricula can help children and adolescents understand the importance of sleep and develop healthy sleep habits from an early age.

Adjusting School Start Times

Adjusting school start times to align with the natural sleep rhythms of adolescents can have significant benefits for students' sleep, academic performance, and overall well-being.

Workplace Initiatives for Better Sleep

Workplace initiatives can also have a significant impact on sleep health. Employers have a role to play in promoting sleep-friendly environments and policies.

Flexibility and Work-Life Balance

Policies that promote flexibility and work-life balance can help employees get adequate sleep. This includes flexible start times, breaks for rest, and limits on overtime work.

Sleep-Friendly Workplace Environments

Creating a sleep-friendly workplace environment, such as providing areas for rest and relaxation and educating employees about the importance of sleep, can improve employee well-being and productivity.

Technology and Sleep Education

Technology can be leveraged to enhance sleep education and promote better sleep habits.

Online Platforms and Apps

Online platforms and apps can provide accessible resources for sleep education. This includes information on sleep hygiene, guided relaxation exercises, and personalized sleep tracking.

Telehealth for Sleep Disorders

Telehealth services can increase access to sleep specialists, especially in underserved areas, making it easier for individuals to seek help for sleep disorders.

Community-Based Sleep Health Programs

Community-based programs can reach a wider audience, particularly in areas where sleep health is not a common topic of discussion.

Community Workshops and Seminars

Conducting workshops and seminars in community centers, libraries, and other public spaces can spread knowledge about sleep health to diverse populations.

Collaborations with Healthcare Providers

Collaborating with healthcare providers to incorporate sleep health into routine care can help in early identification and management of sleep disorders.

Global Sleep Health Initiatives

Given the universality of sleep, global initiatives can play a crucial role in addressing sleep health on a larger scale.

International Collaborations

Collaborations between countries and international health organizations can lead to the development of global guidelines and strategies for sleep health.

Addressing Cultural Differences

Global initiatives should also consider cultural differences in sleep practices and attitudes, tailoring programs to fit various cultural contexts.

Conclusion

Public health initiatives and education about sleep are vital in addressing the widespread issue of sleep deprivation and promoting better sleep habits. By integrating sleep into health policies, educational curricula, workplace practices, and community programs, we can create a more sleep-aware society.

Conclusion

Summarizing the Key Insights

In "Dreaming of Youth," we have journeyed through the multi-faceted world of sleep, exploring its profound impact on health, aging, and well-being. This conclusion aims to encapsulate the key insights gleaned from the book, highlighting the crucial role sleep plays in our lives.

The Fundamental Nature of Sleep

One of the most fundamental insights of the book is the understanding that sleep is a vital, yet often neglected, component of health. It's not just a passive state but a dynamic process crucial for the body's repair, restoration, and rejuvenation. The quality and quantity of our sleep directly influence our physical, cognitive, and emotional health.

Sleep's Impact on Physical Health

The book underscores the significant impact of sleep on physical health. From its role in bolstering the immune system to its influence on metabolic and cardiovascular health, sleep is shown to be a cornerstone of physical well-being. The relationship between sleep and chronic conditions like obesity, diabetes, and heart disease highlights the necessity of adequate and quality sleep for disease prevention and management.

Cognitive and Emotional Aspects of Sleep

Sleep's influence extends to cognitive and emotional dimensions of health. It plays a vital role in memory consolidation, learning, and cognitive processing. The book also delves into the emotional aspects, illustrating how sleep affects mood, stress management, and mental health. The connection between sleep and disorders like depression and anxiety emphasizes the need for good sleep to maintain emotional and psychological well-being.

The Challenge of Sleep Disorders

Addressing various sleep disorders, the book sheds light on their prevalence and impact on health and longevity. From insomnia and sleep apnea to restless legs syndrome and narcolepsy, these conditions are explored with an emphasis on their diagnosis, management, and treatment. The book advocates for a greater awareness and understanding of these disorders as critical to enhancing sleep quality and overall health.

The Influence of Diet, Exercise, and Lifestyle

"Dreaming of Youth" highlights the significant influence of diet, exercise, and lifestyle choices on sleep quality. It promotes the idea that healthy eating habits, regular physical activity, and balanced lifestyle choices are pivotal in improving sleep. The book suggests practical changes and interventions that can be incorporated into daily routines to foster better sleep.

Technological Advancements in Sleep

The exploration of technological advancements in sleep science and their applications is another key insight. From wearables and apps for sleep tracking to innovative treatments and therapies, the book delves into how technology is shaping our understanding and management of sleep. It also cautions against over-reliance on technology, advocating for a balanced approach.

Cultural and Societal Perspectives

Understanding global sleep patterns and cultural attitudes towards sleep is crucial, as highlighted in the book. It explores how cultural norms, societal pressures, and lifestyle differences across the world influence sleep habits and attitudes. The book argues for the importance of recognizing and respecting these cultural differences in sleep practices.

Public Health and Sleep Education

The book emphasizes the role of public health initiatives and education in promoting sleep awareness and healthy sleep practices. It advocates for integrating sleep education into public health policies, school curricula, and workplace health programs. The book underscores the necessity of collective efforts in addressing the widespread issue of sleep deprivation.

The Future of Sleep Research

Looking forward, "Dreaming of Youth" paints an optimistic picture of the future of sleep research. The potential for new discoveries and advancements that could further our understanding of sleep and its relationship with aging and health is highlighted. The book encourages continued research and innovation in the field of sleep science.

Conclusion

In essence, this book serves as an introductory guide, offering insights into the complex world of sleep and its myriad connections to our daily lives. It underscores the critical role of sleep in maintaining health and vitality, particularly as we age. By weaving together scientific research, practical advice, and cultural perspectives, the book provides a holistic view of sleep and its indispensable role in our journey towards a healthier, more vibrant life.

Final Thoughts

As we conclude "Dreaming of Youth," it becomes evident that sleep is not merely a passive state of rest. Instead, it emerges as a fundamental pillar of health and vitality, particularly in the context of aging. This final chapter reflects on the critical role of sleep in the aging process and emphasizes the importance of embracing it for a healthier and more fulfilling life.

Sleep: A Key to Healthy Aging

The journey through "Dreaming of Youth" has illuminated the intricate ways in which sleep impacts every aspect of our health as we age. From supporting physical well-being to maintaining cognitive functions and emotional balance, sleep proves to be an indispensable ally.

Physical Restoration and Disease Prevention

As we age, the restorative power of sleep plays a crucial role in physical health. It helps in repairing the body, bolstering the immune system, and reducing the risk of age-related diseases. Quality sleep is associated with a lower risk of developing chronic conditions like heart disease, diabetes, and obesity.

Cognitive Maintenance and Mental Health

Sleep's influence on cognitive health is profound. Adequate sleep aids in memory consolidation, supports learning, and preserves cognitive functions, which are particularly crucial as we age. Furthermore, sleep's role in emotional regulation and mental health cannot be overstated, with good sleep hygiene linked to lower risks of depression and anxiety.

Challenges in Maintaining Sleep Quality with Age

Despite its importance, maintaining sleep quality often becomes more challenging as we age. Changes in sleep patterns, the prevalence of sleep disorders, and age-related health issues can make achieving restful sleep difficult. However, understanding these challenges is the first step in overcoming them.

Adapting to Changes in Sleep Patterns

Adapting to changes in sleep patterns is key. This might involve adjusting daily routines or seeking medical advice for sleep disturbances. It's crucial to recognize and adapt to these changes rather than accept poor sleep as an inevitable part of aging.

Addressing Sleep Disorders Proactively

Proactively addressing sleep disorders can significantly improve quality of life in later years. Whether it's consulting sleep specialists for conditions like sleep apnea or incorporating relaxation techniques for insomnia, taking active steps to manage sleep issues is essential.

Embracing a Holistic Approach to Sleep

Embracing sleep as a pillar of health requires a holistic approach, integrating various aspects of lifestyle, from diet and exercise to stress management and mental health.

Lifestyle Modifications

Lifestyle modifications such as a balanced diet, regular physical activity, and stress reduction can enhance sleep quality. Creating a sleep-conducive environment and maintaining a regular sleep schedule are also pivotal.

The Role of Technology and Mindfulness

While technology offers tools for monitoring and improving sleep, it's important to use these aids mindfully. Techniques like meditation and mindfulness can also play a significant role in preparing the mind and body for restful sleep.

The Societal and Cultural Dimensions of Sleep

Recognizing the societal and cultural dimensions of sleep is crucial. Societal attitudes towards work, leisure, and health invariably affect how we sleep. Advocating for healthier work-life balances and greater public awareness about the importance of sleep can shift societal norms towards more sleep-friendly practices.

Global Perspectives on Sleep

Understanding and respecting global perspectives on sleep can also offer valuable insights into diverse approaches to rest and rejuvenation. Different cultures can provide alternative viewpoints and practices that might enrich our own sleep habits.

The Future of Sleep in Aging

Looking towards the future, the continued evolution of sleep science promises deeper insights into the relationship between sleep and aging. This ongoing research will be vital in developing more effective strategies for enhancing sleep in our later years.

Innovations in Sleep Research and Medicine

Innovations in sleep research and medicine could lead to new treatments for sleep disorders and more personalized approaches to sleep health. This holds the promise of better sleep quality for older adults, contributing to longer and healthier lives.

Conclusion

In essence, embracing sleep as a cornerstone of health and vitality is a critical aspect of aging gracefully. This book serves not just as a guide to better sleep but as an invitation to reevaluate and prioritize this fundamental aspect of our lives. By doing so, we open the door to not only extended longevity but also a higher quality of life, filled with vitality, clarity, and emotional balance. Sleep, therefore, should be cherished and nurtured as a precious resource, a true companion through the journey of aging.

Appendix A: Resources for further reading and research

The journey through "Dreaming of Youth" provides an overview of the multifaceted nature of sleep and its impact on health and aging. However, the exploration of sleep does not end with this book. For those seeking to delve deeper into the subject, the world of sleep science and health offers a vast reservoir of resources. This appendix is dedicated to guiding readers toward further reading and research in the field of sleep.

Academic Journals and Publications

The field of sleep science is continually evolving, with new research and findings frequently published. Academic journals and publications are excellent sources for the latest research and in-depth analysis.

"Sleep" Journal

Published by the Sleep Research Society, this peer-reviewed journal offers a range of articles on sleep studies, including the latest research findings, reviews, and clinical trials.

"Journal of Sleep Research"

This journal provides a platform for research on sleep and its disorders, covering aspects from basic science to clinical applications.

"Journal of Clinical Sleep Medicine"

Published by the American Academy of Sleep Medicine, this journal focuses on clinical studies and reviews related to sleep medicine, an invaluable resource for those interested in clinical aspects of sleep.

Books on Sleep Science and Health

Several books offer insightful and accessible information on sleep, ranging from scientific explorations to practical advice.

"Why We Sleep" by Matthew Walker

This book by neuroscientist Matthew Walker is a comprehensive guide to the science of sleep, exploring its importance for health, brain function, and psychological well-being.

"The Sleep Solution" by W. Chris Winter

Written by a sleep specialist, this book offers practical advice for overcoming common sleep problems and improving sleep health.

"The Promise of Sleep" by William C. Dement

This book delves into the science of sleep and its role in our lives, written by one of the pioneers in sleep research.

Online Resources and Websites

The internet offers a plethora of resources on sleep, from educational websites to online courses.

National Sleep Foundation

The National Sleep Foundation's website provides a wealth of information on sleep health, disorders, and tips for better sleep.

Sleep Education

A website run by the American Academy of Sleep Medicine, offering resources, research updates, and educational content on sleep.

Coursera and edX

Online educational platforms like Coursera and edX offer courses on sleep science and health, taught by experts in the field.

Sleep Tracking and Analysis Tools

For those interested in monitoring their own sleep patterns, various tools and apps are available.

Sleep Cycle App

This app analyzes sleep patterns and offers insights into sleep quality. It also includes features like sleep notes and a smart alarm.

Fitbit and Other Wearables

Wearable devices like Fitbit provide sleep tracking features, offering data on sleep stages, duration, and quality.

Podcasts on Sleep

Podcasts offer an engaging way to learn about sleep, featuring interviews with experts and discussions on various sleep-related topics.

"Sleepy Time Mumbles"

This podcast discusses various aspects of sleep science in an accessible and engaging manner.

"The Sleep Health Podcast"

Hosted by a sleep physician, this podcast covers a range of topics related to sleep health and disorders.

Support Groups and Forums

For those dealing with sleep disorders or seeking to share experiences and tips, support groups and online forums can be invaluable.

Sleep Apnea Support Forums

Online forums for sleep apnea patients offer a platform for sharing experiences, advice, and support.

Insomnia Support Groups

Support groups for insomnia can be found both online and in local communities, providing a space for sharing coping strategies and support.

Conclusion

The pursuit of knowledge about sleep is an ongoing journey. The resources listed here offer just a starting point for further exploration into the complex and fascinating world of sleep. Whether through academic research, books, online courses, or community forums, continuing to learn about sleep can enrich one's understanding and contribute to better sleep health.

Appendix B: Sleep assessment tools and questionnaires

Understanding and improving sleep quality is a crucial aspect of maintaining overall health and well-being, particularly as we age. To aid in this process, various sleep assessment tools and questionnaires have been developed. These tools are designed to help individuals and healthcare providers evaluate sleep patterns, identify potential sleep disorders, and monitor the effectiveness of interventions. In this appendix we explore some of the commonly used sleep assessment tools and their applications.

The Role of Sleep Assessment Tools

Sleep assessment tools serve multiple purposes. They can help in self-assessment, aiding individuals in understanding their own sleep patterns and habits. In a clinical setting, these tools assist healthcare providers in diagnosing sleep disorders and tailoring treatment plans. They are essential for capturing the subjective experience of sleep, which might not always be evident in objective measures like polysomnography.

Common Sleep Assessment Questionnaires

Several questionnaires have been developed over the years to assess various aspects of sleep quality and disorders. These tools are often used both in research and clinical practice.

The Pittsburgh Sleep Quality Index (PSQI)

The PSQI is a widely used questionnaire that assesses sleep quality over a one-month period. It includes questions about sleep duration, latency, disturbances, and daytime dysfunction. The PSQI helps in identifying patterns indicative of poor sleep quality.

The Epworth Sleepiness Scale (ESS)

The ESS is a simple, self-administered questionnaire that measures a person's general level of daytime sleepiness. It asks individuals to rate their likelihood of falling asleep in different situations, helping to identify excessive daytime sleepiness, a common symptom of several sleep disorders.

The Insomnia Severity Index (ISI)

The ISI is a brief questionnaire that assesses the nature, severity, and impact of insomnia. It includes questions about sleep onset, maintenance, early morning awakening, and the degree of distress caused by sleep problems.

Tools for Specific Sleep Disorders

Certain tools are specifically designed to assess particular sleep disorders, providing targeted insights.

The Berlin Questionnaire

The Berlin Questionnaire is used to assess the risk of obstructive sleep apnea. It includes questions about snoring, breathing pauses during sleep, and risk factors like hypertension and obesity.

The Restless Legs Syndrome (RLS) Questionnaire

This tool is designed to diagnose RLS, a disorder characterized by an uncontrollable urge to move the legs. It focuses on the presence and severity of leg discomfort and the urge to move, especially in the evening and during rest.

Diaries and Sleep Logs

In addition to structured questionnaires, sleep diaries or logs are a valuable tool for assessing sleep patterns. Individuals record details about their sleep and waking times, sleep quality, and any disturbances they experience. This information can provide a comprehensive view of an individual's sleep habits over time.

Application of Sleep Diaries

Sleep diaries are particularly useful for identifying patterns and behaviors that may contribute to sleep disturbances. They are often used in conjunction with other assessment tools to provide a holistic view of an individual's sleep.

Technological Tools for Sleep Assessment

Advancements in technology have led to the development of various digital tools for sleep assessment.

Wearable Sleep Trackers

Devices like smartwatches and fitness bands can track sleep duration, quality, and stages. While not as accurate as clinical assessments, they provide a convenient way for individuals to monitor their sleep.

Smartphone Sleep Apps

Several smartphone apps offer sleep tracking and analysis features. They use the phone's sensors to monitor movement and estimate sleep patterns, providing users with insights into their sleep quality.

The Importance of Professional Evaluation

While these tools are valuable for initial assessment and self-monitoring, it's important to consult healthcare professionals for a definitive diagnosis and treatment plan, especially when a sleep disorder is suspected. Professionals can interpret the results of these tools within the broader context of an individual's overall health and lifestyle.

Conclusion

Sleep assessment tools and questionnaires play a crucial role in understanding and improving sleep quality. They offer valuable insights for both individuals and healthcare providers, aiding in the identification of sleep issues and the monitoring of treatment effectiveness.

Appendix C: Directory of sleep clinics and experts

Directory of Sleep Clinics and Experts

For individuals seeking professional assistance with sleep-related issues, a directory of sleep clinics and experts can be an invaluable resource. Such a directory provides access to specialized care and expert advice, essential for diagnosing and treating sleep disorders effectively. In the appendices of "Dreaming of Youth," we present a guide to navigating the landscape of sleep clinics and experts, highlighting the importance of seeking professional help when needed.

The Importance of Specialized Sleep Clinics

Sleep clinics play a crucial role in diagnosing and treating sleep disorders. These specialized facilities are equipped with the tools and expertise necessary for comprehensive sleep evaluations, including overnight sleep studies (polysomnography), home sleep apnea testing, and other diagnostic procedures.

Services Offered by Sleep Clinics

Sleep clinics typically offer a range of services, including:

- Diagnosis and treatment of sleep disorders such as insomnia, sleep apnea, restless legs syndrome, and narcolepsy.
- Overnight sleep studies to monitor sleep patterns, breathing, heart rate, and other physiological functions.
- Behavioral therapy and counseling for sleep-related issues.

Finding a Sleep Clinic

When looking for a sleep clinic, there are several factors to consider to ensure you receive high-quality care.

Accreditation and Certification

Choosing a clinic that is accredited by a recognized body, such as the American Academy of Sleep Medicine (AASM) in the United States, ensures that the facility meets specific standards of care and professionalism.

Expertise and Experience

It is important to look into the qualifications and experience of the healthcare professionals working at the clinic. Board-certified sleep medicine doctors and experienced sleep technologists are indicators of a reputable clinic.

Insurance and Cost

Before scheduling an appointment, it's wise to check whether the clinic accepts your health insurance and to understand the costs involved, particularly for procedures like sleep studies.

Sleep Experts and Their Roles

In addition to sleep clinics, there are various sleep experts who play vital roles in managing sleep disorders.

Sleep Medicine Physicians

Sleep medicine physicians are doctors who specialize in diagnosing and treating sleep disorders. They can provide comprehensive care, from initial consultation to treatment and follow-up.

Clinical Psychologists and Therapists

For disorders like insomnia, clinical psychologists or therapists trained in behavioral sleep medicine can be invaluable. They offer therapies like Cognitive Behavioral Therapy for Insomnia (CBT-I), which is highly effective in treating insomnia.

Pulmonologists, Neurologists, and Other Specialists

Some sleep disorders may require the expertise of specialists like pulmonologists (for sleep apnea) or neurologists (for narcolepsy and other neurological sleep disorders).

Online Resources for Locating Sleep Clinics and Experts

There are several online resources that can help in locating sleep clinics and experts.

Professional Organizations

Websites of professional organizations like the American Academy of Sleep Medicine offer directories of accredited sleep centers and certified sleep professionals.

Hospital and Healthcare Systems

Many hospitals and healthcare systems have sleep centers or departments dedicated to sleep medicine. Their websites can provide information on the services offered and the specialists available.

Online Reviews and Ratings

Online platforms where patients review and rate doctors and clinics can offer insights into the experiences of others, although these should be approached with a degree of caution.

The Global Landscape of Sleep Medicine

For those outside the United States, there are numerous international organizations and clinics specializing in sleep medicine.

International Sleep Organizations

Organizations like the World Sleep Society and the European Sleep Research Society provide resources and directories for sleep clinics and experts around the world.

Country-Specific Resources

Many countries have their own sleep medicine societies or associations, which can provide localized information on sleep clinics and experts.

Conclusion

Access to a directory of sleep clinics and experts is a vital resource for anyone experiencing sleep-related issues. Professional evaluation and treatment are crucial for effectively managing sleep disorders and improving overall health and well-being.

www.ingramcontent.com/pod-product-compliance
Lightning Source LLC
Chambersburg PA
CBHW070900260726
48661CB00004B/1520